Advance praise for *Mindful Movement*

Mindful Movement has come along at just the right time. Dr. David Tannenbaum and Risa Sheppard, along with most cutting-edge scientists, have gone beyond the "conventional" thinking that pain, discomfort, and disease are the root issues that need to be cured. This book brings to light that our symptoms are merely warning signs of deeper mind-body imbalances and/or dysfunctions. They offer ways to optimize our health by addressing underlying causes of physical dis-ease that originate in our emotions and mind. In my forty years as a doctor, acknowledging the mind-body connection has been key to promoting health in my practice. Kudos to Risa Sheppard and Dr. Tannenbaum for showing us how to address the causes of pain and dis-ease so that symptoms do not need to manifest themselves. **Dr. Ron Oberstein, president of Life Chiropractic College West**

I have known and worked with Risa Sheppard over the years since she first came to Ron Fletchers Pilates studio in 1975. This book that she and Dr. Tannenbaum have written, *Mindful Movement*, is an excellent source of guidance to a pain-free life, integrating body and mind. I know from experience that it works! **Katherine Ross, Academy Award-nominated and Golden Globe Award-winning actress**

Dr. Tannenbaum is a miracle worker. He has made my life better, healthier, and happier. I am so glad that he has teamed with Risa Sheppard to give us *Mindful Movement*. I urge you to read their book. **Debra Messing, Emmy Award-winning actress**

There are three very important things in my life:

1. My faith in God.
2. I have been blessed to have a wonderful instructor, Risa Sheppard, who has guided me through the steps of Pilates. Pilates strengthens my core to help the rest of the body follow suit.
3. Maintaining chiropractic work on my body.

Thank you, Risa Sheppard, for what you have done to guide me in the art of Pilates. I know that your new book written with Dr. Tannenbaum, *Mindful Movement*, will help so many. **Reba McEntire, country singer, songwriter, and actress**

As I look back on my ninety-five years on this planet, I find that it has been a continuous acquisition of knowledge.

- I learned how to cope and meet life's challenges head-on.

- I learned from my husband, Jack LaLanne, that exercise and proper nutrition can help reverse the aging process

- I learned from Dr. William Hornaday [and] Drs. Frank and Anita Richelieu the teachings of Ernest Holmes, Science of Mind and Spiritual Living. Both Jack and I believed that everything starts in the mind.

- I learned (Jack had a chiropractic degree) how chiropractic can help keep your body and spine aligned.

- I learned about and tried all kinds of therapy and found that through searching you can find one that helps and fits your need.

Risa and I have similar teachings. She embodies meeting life's challenges through exercise and nutrition. She is a student and teacher of Science of Mind and is sought by many to lecture on BAM (Body and Mind) Therapy. Risa's collaboration with chiropractor and co-author Dr. David Tannenbaum has led to this wonderful new book, *Mindful Movement*. I highly recommend you take to heart their wisdom for living a higher quality life. **Elaine LaLanne, health and fitness author and widow of Jack LaLanne**

MINDFUL *Movement*

MINDFUL *Movement*

Heal
Your
Back
Pain
with
BAM THERAPY

DR. DAVID TANNENBAUM D.C.
& RISA SHEPPARD

NEWMAN SPRINGS PUBLISHING
320 Broad Street
Red Bank, NJ 07701

First originally published by Newman Springs Publishing 2023

ISBN 979-8-88763-232-2 (Paperback)
ISBN 979-8-88763-233-9 (Digital)

Contents

Introduction to BAM Therapy

We live in a new age of health care. More and more science-based healing modalities accept that there is a profound mind-body-spirit connection and that it is not strange to utilize therapies that rely on psychological and spiritual practices to deal with pain. There is a growing field of somatic therapies that start from the clear understanding that our spiritual and mental states are connected to our sense of body wellness. Some popular somatic therapies are sensorimotor psychotherapy,[1] the Hakomi Method,[2] bioenergetic analysis,[3] and biodynamic psychotherapy.[4]

Somatic therapies differ from BAM Therapy in that they have a direct focus on mental and emotional health issues that are addressed through dance, breath work, and meditation. As you will learn, BAM Therapy touches on these methods, but our focus is rooted in our combined healing experiences of many years of chiropractic and Pilates body-based understanding of healing. We may begin with the body, but BAM Therapy simultaneously addresses the mental and spiritual

---

1   Sensorimotor psychotherapy is a modality developed by Dr. Pat Ogden, founder of the Sensorimotor Psychotherapy Institute. For more information, see https://sensorimotorpsychotherapy.org/.

2   The Hakomi Method is a modality developed by Ron Kurtz. For more information, see https://hakomiinstitute.com/.

3   Bioenergetic analysis is an approach to therapy that focuses on the energy between the body and mind. For more information, see United States Association for Body Psychotherapy at https://usabp.org/.

4   Biodynamic psychotherapy is a therapy that emphasizes the body's role in psychotherapy. For more information, see Institute of Biodynamic Medicine, https://biodynamic.org/what-is/biodynamic-psychotherapy/.

dimensions of the person seeking healing. Our work has been profoundly guided by such mind-body-spirit pioneers as Louise Hay, Joe Pilates, and Ernest Holmes.

Between us, we have been practicing our techniques for more than seventy years. We started collaborating around 2000, having met through a mutual friend who thought we would work well together.

In 2006, Risa was diagnosed with a benign tumor called acoustic neuroma. She experienced intense headaches and dizziness and decided to have an MRI to detect the source of her pain. The imaging revealed an inner ear tumor that had grown so big that it had started pressing against her brain. Despite this discovery, Risa continued working, but she eventually had to go to the hospital and have the tumor removed.

Risa's anticipated five-day hospital stay turned into a month because of complications. A second surgery was done to drain the buildup of fluid in her brain. When a shunt was inserted, she lost all of her hearing and the use of the balance nerve on the right side of her face. After six months of rehabilitation, she was able to get back to work. Risa's experience brought home to her how precious life is, and she wanted to make a difference in the lives of those who suffer from chronic pain.

Risa's doctors were amazed at how fast she healed. She said the healing happened because of her years of doing Pilates, receiving chiropractic care, and daily use of positive affirmations.

David was born and raised on the East Coast, in suburban New Jersey, just outside of Manhattan. He suffered from chronic asthma, and at a young age, he hurt his back when playing basketball. He could not walk as a result of this lower back injury. His mom took him to several specialists, but no one could figure out what was wrong with him.

David's dad, who was a health fanatic in the 1970s, took him to a chiropractor. The doctor x-rayed his back and showed him where the disc problem was—at his lower lumbar L4. The chiropractor gave David an adjustment, and he was able to walk out of the office. He continued the chiropractic treatments.

One day, David's mom noticed that he no longer needed his inhaler for asthma, and she asked him why. It was clear to David that the regular chiropractic care and adjustments had helped free up the nerve supply to his lungs. His asthma was gone.

From this teenage experience, David decided he wanted to help people get well from acute and chronic issues without drugs or surgery. He attended chiropractic school in Atlanta when he was quite young; in fact, he was the youngest in his class.

David found chiropractic training interesting because so many of his fellow students had similar issues that had been cleared up by getting adjusted. They, too, had been inspired to become chiropractic healers because of their experiences.

One year, on a trip to California to see some of his colleagues in the heart of winter, he couldn't believe how beautiful, warm, and progressive Los Angeles was. Upon returning to New Jersey, he sold his practice and home and moved to Southern California. In his thirty-plus years of practice in Los Angeles, David has been honored to bring healing to some of the biggest names in the film, music, and sports worlds. He had never imagined that a kid from New Jersey would one day make a difference in so many people's lives.

Once our paths crossed and we became close friends and colleagues, we joined forces to create BAM Therapy which, in turn, led us to write this book. We want to share our years of experience and our techniques with a bigger audience around the world.

Everybody knows that stress can cause illness. Some of the most common ailments we typically think of as the result of stress include ulcers, migraines, heart conditions, and cancer. Recent medical research has shown that emotional stress, particularly from fear and anger, is the trigger for most health issues, including common pain-related syndromes.

Science of Mind and Pilates, Risa Sheppard

I have been interested in and involved with Pilates and the world of metaphysics (beyond the physical senses) since the 1970s. I have always been a searcher for the meaning of life and my part in it. I have always felt there is something else, some higher intelligence much greater than mine or anyone else's. I don't believe that this crazy, beautiful, war-torn world filled with strife and disappointment is all there is. There must be something more, something we can attach ourselves to that will make sense of it all and allow us to reveal our own bliss.

This may be the reason I was so attracted to and taken by Pilates. This practice showed me a new way to move my body and connect with my spirit. It gave me the freedom of expression and a way to overcome the prohibitions of bodily limitations, and it allowed me to feel an exhilaration I had never experienced.

Interestingly, I came across Science of Mind—the melding of philosophy, religion, and science—and Pilates at nearly the same time, in 1975.[5] I had just graduated from the University of California, Los Angeles. I wanted to be a film star, but I also needed to make money. We baby boomers were taught to fend for ourselves, and as children of children of the Great Depression, our parents taught us the tough way to grow up. Nothing was given to us. We had to appreciate all that we had and work for everything we wanted. That

---

5   Adapted from "What is Science of Mind" in the Scottsdale Science of Mind website: https://scottsdalecsl.org/what-is-science-of-mind/.

Science of Mind was developed in the early twentieth century by writer and philosopher Ernest Holmes. Dr. Holmes studied the world's religious traditions and the sacred writings of the ancient Greek philosophers to the then present-day spiritual and religious leaders and found common ideas and spiritual truths in all. He taught that the Universal Spirit—God—is the source of all things, that this one power moves through us as love and creativity, and that we can actively participate with it to create happier, fulfilling, peaceful, and joyous lives.

Here is an excerpt from an Ernest Holmes's paper describing the Science of Mind:

The Science of Mind is built on the theory that there is One Infinite Mind which of necessity includes all that is, whether it be the intelligence in man, the life in the animal, or the invisible Presence which is God. In it we learn to have a spiritual sense of things. This spiritual sense of things is what is meant by the Consciousness of Christ. To be able to discern the spiritual idea back of its physical symbol is to use the mind that Jesus used.

The Science of Mind is intensely practical because it teaches us how to use the Mind Principle for definite purposes, such as helping those who are sick, impoverished, or unhappy. Each one of us should learn to become a practitioner of this science, a demonstrator of its Principle, a conscious user of its Power. Power already exists, but the existence of Power is of no particular value to us until we use it. We must not only be conscious of Power, but we must be actively conscious of it. This is one of the first lessons we learn in the Science of Mind.

way, if the economy failed, the world collapsed, or the sky fell, we could still make it through to the next day.

It is true that some came through those times unscathed, like a ninety-year-old client of mine who recently said, "I didn't even know there was a depression." But for most of us and our parents, earning a living and surviving meant we had to be smart, clever, and gutsy. I can honestly say that I have my fair share of those attributes. Despite insecurities, a fear of abandonment, being a people pleaser, and wanting worldwide recognition—for what, I will never know—I was determined to be successful.

But I needed help. My childhood home life was not religious. Both my parents were Catholic, but they wanted their children to find their own religion. I longed for answers to life's big questions like "What's it all about?" and, importantly, "How can I get there faster?" I was a young girl wanting to be an actress in Hollywood, and I needed guidance.

Science of Mind was established in 1927 by Dr. Ernest Holmes. It is a spiritual, philosophical, and metaphysical religious teaching and community within the New Thought movement. Dr. Holmes developed the Science of Mind philosophy to show how the inner experience of God gives entry to the power of God. Changing the way we think about our conditions causes the power of the universe to change those conditions to make our lives better. Science of Mind identifies the spiritual principles that apply equally to everyone in every situation, and it teaches us how to use them to our advantage.

Mental health experts have significantly underestimated the importance of lifestyle factors as contributors to physical, emotional, behavioral, and spiritual pathologies. Mind-body techniques have been underused even though such techniques have minimal risks and significant benefits.

Pilates is an exercise method developed in Germany by Joseph Pilates at the beginning of the last century. Here I found a physical expression that captured my heart. I felt like a dancer without being a dancer. Pilates teaches grace, control, mindfulness of the body temple, and a life free of strife, illness, or pain of any kind—sensations that all humans want to feel.

I learned that I could go within, find that perfect place, and allow my mind to connect with my body. I found the power within me, and it was far greater than I could have imagined. From that point on, I competed only with myself and strived to be better each day. Sometimes I hit the mark, and sometimes I do not. But there is always tomorrow. Starting over where we are is a sure sign that we are going to be and do better. Pilates forces us to go within, find our own rhythm, and create a physical sensation that is uniquely our own.

I believe Pilates is about personal responsibility. It gives us the feeling of control over our own existence but not just for the time that we are learning and performing the movements. This is because it is *movement* that is essential in life. Not being or feeling is stagnating. It is death. Movement is life, and we all love to move.

Movement with Pilates helps us strive to improve, constantly move beyond our limitations to discover something more, and be satisfied with who we are at the present moment. We make mistakes and learn from them. We are totally involved in the moment, without competition from others. We do not try to be smarter, fitter, or happier than anyone else. A tall order? Yes, but in movement with Pilates, we move to our own rhythm, our own pace, and our own ideal of personal perfection.

I see life goals through the teachings of Pilates: freedom of the body, control of the mind, and unique expression of our own spirits. Movement is expressing fully that which is within us always: perfection, wholeness, and completion. We may not do a movement perfectly, but there is a perfect movement within each and every one of us yearning to be expressed.

Science of Mind showed me a new way of seeing things with teachings that made sense even as they challenged me, such as "Change your thinking spiritually, and your life will change" and "You'll find your true path, whatever that is." These were not the answers I was looking for, but I now had a dawning sense that there was something larger than my little ego that I should be aiming for, something else that wanted to act on the screen. In short, I began to know that there was something more to living a full life—and I was determined to find it.

Something about Science of Mind's message rang true. I started going to church regularly, took classes, and continued to see my Science of Mind spiritual counselor.

I was finding meaning in what I was doing. I began to take responsibility for myself. I was doing everything the church and the philosophy told me to do to be a happier and more fulfilled woman. And it was working.

Over the next forty-plus years, I developed my Pilates career by using the principles of Science of Mind as a touchstone. I created a unique form of Pilates now known around the world as the Sheppard Method. I believe that if it were not for my application of the Science of Mind principles combined with the application of the Pilates principles, I would not be the healthy, vital, youthful, and energetic sixty-five-year-old woman I am today.

In her book *Heal Your Body*, Louise Hay writes, "Both the good in our lives and the dis-ease are the results of mental thought patterns which form our experiences." In other words, for every effect in our lives, there is a thought pattern that precedes and then maintains it. Hayes goes on to say that metaphysical causations describe the power in the words and thoughts that create experiences. There is an awareness of the connection between thoughts, the different parts of the body, and physical problems.

When a part of their body is in dysfunction, often, one of the first things people say is, "If only I knew what was causing this pain!" We run to doctors, physical therapists, and others to solve the problem, but what we don't realize is that untying the mental knot causing the pain is just as important as untying the physical knot. It is only by addressing the mental stressors that we can hope to completely eradicate the symptoms. We may feel better after we have seen a doctor, but the symptoms will often rear their ugly heads again and again if we do not get at the true mental cause.

Scientific research has shown that various emotions and stress factors are stored in different parts of the body. For example, if there is stiffness in your shoulders and neck, you might want to examine whether you are holding any stress factors that are making you unable to move out of the condition. Most of the time, we are not aware of how the mental thought patterns we have held all our lives affect us. But they do.

I am not a psychologist. It is not the objective of this book to delve into your past and uncover traumas. However, as a metaphysical healer, my goal is to help you look within and permanently release and erase the thinking that has prompted your condition. We don't have to know what the thought is or what the trauma was. The higher intelligence within each one of us knows, and by simply declaring with conviction that it holds no power and is no longer effective, we can help release the knot.

In my professional life as a Pilates instructor, I have combined the best of Science of Mind—the scientific and spiritual way of directing the mind and spirit toward a specific goal—and the art of Pilates, as taught to me through first-generation teacher Ron Fletcher. Together, these ideas bring us to the highest level we can be in mind, body, and spirit. It is my joy to be joining Dr. Tannenbaum to share this material with you in *Mindful Movement*.

Chiropractic Care, David Tannenbaum, DC

In my thirty-plus years of practice, I have had a multitude of patients come to me to eliminate their chronic pain. Most have exhausted all Western techniques of healing, from injections to surgery. I have a natural affinity toward people, and I love seeing them rehabilitate themselves in a positive and holistic manner. I have built my practice out of love for others, and I enjoy the process of healing from the inside out.

When Risa first came to me, she was already a seasoned and highly regarded Pilates instructor with a spiritual orientation grounded in her study of Science of Mind. We found that her system of corrective exercise and my chiropractic care were wonderfully compatible. The nervous system is where a lot of memories, trauma, and injury are held. Chiropractic heals the nervous system by removing the pressure in the spine so the body can heal itself naturally. Pilates heals by increasing the body's core strength with a focus on the abdominal muscles, lower back, and buttocks.

But between our two practices, something was missing. We needed a third component. That missing part was the spiritual and emotional aspect of the innermost being and is behind every single factor of pain. For every effect, there is a cause; that is simple science. Together, Risa and I felt we could achieve success. We knew it would take practice and the willingness to see beyond the obvious to delve deep into the subconscious and discover the thought patterns and belief systems that were causing pain.

Chiropractic is the largest, most natural healing profession in the world today that does not incorporate the use of drugs. I have had the incredible opportunity of treating some of the most influential artists and athletes in the world, and I know that no one is immune to pain. No one escapes their unique early childhood belief system that caused them pain and suffering.

BAM Therapy is designed to bring to the surface physical, emotional, and spiritual aspects of a person's life and pain.

It provides a means to make one aware of all the components that go into a fully functioning mind, body, and spirit.

Pain does not need to be a way of life. With BAM Therapy, Risa and I offer a new and exciting way of understanding what may be the underlying cause of your pain. Let us explore the possibilities of how you can increase your joy here on this planet.

PART 1

Stress and the Body

CHAPTER 1

How the Physical Body Reacts to Emotional Stress

*Our anxiety does not come from thinking about
the future, but from wanting to control it.*
-Kahlil Gibran

Stress is a universal aspect of human life. It happens to everyone in the normal course of living. Stress is a sense of emotional or physical tension. Stress strikes us from here, there, and everywhere. It can be caused by events such as an accident or a relationship conflict; or it can come from a thought that makes us feel angry, frustrated, anxious, or nervous. In short, to live is to experience stress.

A helpful definition of stress is attributed to psychologist Richard S. Lazarus. He notes that stress is a condition or feeling experienced when a person perceives that "demands exceed the personal and social resources the individual is able to mobilize." In less formal terms, we feel stressed when circumstances and events feel out of our control.

It is common knowledge that emotions, thoughts, and feelings germinate within the body and manifest in a myriad of ways throughout our lives. Disease, illness, and physical pain can be associated with prior emotional trauma.

Dr. Susanne Babbel, a psychologist specializing in trauma and depression, writes, "Studies have shown that chronic pain might not only be caused by physical injury but also by stress and emotional issues." She further notes that "often, physical pain functions to warn a person that there is still emotional work to be done."[6]

Many people don't think about their inner emotional life and how it can cause physical ailments, except for perhaps the connection between anxiety and ulcers. However, the link between emotional suffering and physical pain is being studied and understood more and more. With an understanding of the connection between emotional stress and physical pain, you can take control and heal yourself through our BAM techniques.

Dr. Murray Grossan of the Grossan Institute writes, "The first thing about healing an illness is to stop the stress and anxiety chemicals that impair normal healing."[7]

Types of Stress

Stress arises through work, family, interaction with day-to-day acts (e.g., driving, shopping, school, or being late for an appointment), forgetting a phone or wallet, and on and on. Some people stress more over small things than big things.

Physical stress can result from an illness or accident. Emotional stress can cause fear, which can jeopardize the immune system. Fear can be in the body from childhood

---

6   Susanne Babbel, MFT, PhD, "The Connections Between Emotional Stress, Trauma and Physical Pain," *Psychology Today* (April 2010).

7   Murray Grossan, "Welcome to the Grossan Institute," The Grossan Institute, http://www.grossaninstitute.com/. (April 27, 2021).

as a result of experiencing death, family financial insecurity, family conflicts, and school pressures.

To begin addressing the consequences of stress, it is helpful to put the causes of stress into two categories: acute and chronic.

Acute stress. Acute stress is short-term stress that goes away quickly. It is caused by minor daily occurrences such as being mad at your spouse for their habits and actions, frustration over a rude person at the store, and so on. Acute stress helps you manage dangerous situations. It also occurs when you do something new or exciting. You feel it when, for example, something or someone suddenly moves toward you, when you have a fight with your coworker or friend, or when you are doing physical activity that demands strength and agility. All people have acute stress at one time or another.

Say you sprained your ankle. You experience not only the pain of the sprain but also an accompanying mental-emotional impact. You now feel clumsy and embarrassed by the fall. Perhaps you fell in childhood, and kids laughed at you, causing embarrassment. This new injury has conjured up that old insecurity.

Mind-body treatment addresses this aspect of acute stress. You could use an affirmation to treat it: "My ankle is strong. The swelling is there for protection. My ankle is protected by the spirit within me. I release anything from my past that makes me feel clumsy. I am standing strong on my two feet, and I am supported in mind, body, and spirit." For anything that might come up, you could use this affirmation: "My ankle is strong. My balance is good. There is no fear in my consciousness, and the healing has taken place right here and right now." Keep affirming that the ankle is whole and healed even before it is completely healed.

Chronic stress. Chronic stress is stress that lasts for a longer period of time and is caused by longtime challenges. It can happen because of financial pressures; poor health; negative family dynamics; or, as we are experiencing at the time of this writing, when dealing with a worldwide pandemic, which has been causing stress from many angles. Any type of stress that goes on for weeks or months is chronic stress. We can become so used to chronic stress that we don't realize it is a problem. If we don't find ways to manage chronic stress, it is likely to lead to health problems.

Stress is different for everyone. It is a state of mental or emotional strain or tension resulting from adverse or highly demanding circumstances—in other words, life. How we deal with life and the inevitability of stressors shows up in the body through physical symptoms and illnesses if we don't deal with its causes.

The Relationship between Stress, Pain, and Disease

Stress is the body's natural and healthy reaction to a challenge or demand. Our bodies react to stress by releasing hormones. These hormones make the brain more alert, cause the muscles to tense, and increase the pulse. In the short term, these reactions are good because they can help us handle the situation causing stress. They are the body's way of protecting itself.

When you have chronic stress, your body stays alert even when there is no danger. Long-term stress puts you at risk for many serious physical and mental health problems, such as the following:

- High blood pressure
- Heart disease
- Diabetes
- Obesity
- Depression
- Anxiety
- Skin problems such as acne and eczema
- Menstrual problems
- Psoriasis
- Headaches
- Allergies
- Shortness of breath
- Back pain
- Muscle pain
- Dizziness
- Stomach troubles including irritable bowel syndrome

Taking a stress test is one way to assess the degree of stress you live with. There are a number of stress tests available, from one-on-one sessions with your psychologist to online tests. A popular test anyone can take to get a sense of how stress may be impacting their life is the Holmes and

Rahe Stress Scale.[8] In 1967, psychiatrists Thomas Holmes and Richard Rahe studied whether or not stress contributes to illness. They surveyed more than five thousand medical patients and asked them to state whether they had experienced any of forty-three specific life events in the previous two years.

Each event, called a Life Change Unit, has a specific rating for stress levels. The more events the patient experienced, the higher the score. The higher the score and the higher the rating of each event, the more likely the patient was to become ill.

Taking such a test can help you to identify and reduce the stressors in your life.

Your Quest for Better Health

As a Pilates expert and a chiropractic doctor, we choose to begin our quest for better health with the spine. The spine is our life support from the moment of birth. It represents and coincides with many aspects of pain and suffering.

The information in the following chapters will give you insights into your own thought processes that may have contributed to your particular pain. "It's the mind itself which shapes the body," says Joseph Pilates.

Ernest Holmes, the founder of Science of Mind, believed that where your mind goes, energy flows.

We will explore this idea in the pages to follow. The aim is to help you examine the thoughts you have that may contribute to your particular pain.

---

8   You can take the Holmes and Rahe Stress scale at the website of The American Institute of Stress at www.stress.org/holmes-rahe-stress-inventory.

We will explore "the mental thought patterns that form our experience," as Religious Science teacher and best-selling author Louise Hay writes in her award-winning book *Heal Your Body*. Much of my (Risa) inspiration comes from the years I personally studied the Religious Science metaphysical healing practice and the numerous clients I have worked with since 1975.

Simply stated, it is your thought that creates your reality. Change your thoughts, and you change your life. Easier said than done. Believe me; we know. We are all used to thinking in a particular way, and changing our perceptions seems impossible. But it is not impossible; actually, it is quite easy. However, it takes intelligence and discipline. If you are reading this book, you are already intelligent and disciplined, so I know we are moving together in the right direction!

When someone comes to me with back pain, I listen to them discuss where it hurts, when the pain started, and what was going on in their life at the time. If there is a pinched nerve in the neck region, I know that this region has to do with looking at all sides of a situation. I ask the client if they had any experience in their life where they didn't understand or appreciate another person's idea of a situation or when and where they were unwilling to turn their head and look the other way. Perhaps their stiff neck or the pinched nerve in their neck would release with the proper physical therapy (Pilates or chiropractic treatment) coupled with right thinking.

I would start with a "spiritual mind treatment." This process is a scientific way of adjusting the mind to think of the positive—an outcome we envision and want.

There is a specific way that we as health-care providers approach a spiritual mind treatment. Let's call it a scientific prayer, one that realigns thought patterns with the divine universal medium. Some people call it God, others the universe, and still others the spirit. The terminology does not matter. We only need to know we are in charge of our own lives and that we have power over it all. Note that this is not an absolute statement. We don't have power over all that happens to us. We cannot stop the COVID-19 pandemic that surrounds us, for example. But we do have power over how to respond to whatever comes our way.

The spirit maintains us and is with us in our hearts at all times, and we have access to this higher power. BAM Therapy offers you tools and a process to quickly and effectively rid yourself of unwanted and self-destructive thought patterns, which, in turn, will help transform and heal whatever malady you have.

We offer you new ways of thinking about your current situation. You will learn spiritual mind treatments that are sure to help you think and move differently. You will also receive tools to realign your true self with what you want to experience.

CHAPTER 2

BAM Therapy

But one had to go back to the beginning of things, always.
Trace the thread of life—find the knot—untangle it.
-Martha Ostenso

Today, the number one ailment affecting Americans is back pain, which impacts 60 to 80 percent of the population. In addition, nearly 70 million adults suffer from arthritis, making it the leading cause of disability. Traditional medicine treats these common pain syndromes as mechanical problems to be cured by mechanical means. But if new research is true and these problems have more to do with people's feelings, personalities, and lives, then the conventional management of these pain syndromes is clearly inadequate.

The Orthopedic Clinic of North America did research on the aftermath of patients who underwent back surgery and found some alarming statistics. The overall failure rate of back surgery patients was between 20 and 40 percent. We think this is because traditional medicine focuses on the mechanics of the body, while the real problem appears to relate more to what makes the body machine work: the mind.

Today, many are dissatisfied with traditional medical treatments and the trauma of conventional surgery. This has created a multibillion-dollar worldwide market niche for an integrated treatment method that combines spiritual and emotional therapies with quality pain management.

We created BAM Therapy to fulfill this need. It is a step-by-step self-treatment program to promote wellness and healing for common ailments. BAM Therapy has been used to successfully treat thousands of people with ailments such as chronic back pain, headaches, arthritis, and digestive issues.

What we have set out to accomplish with BAM Therapy is to untie the mental knots along with the physical knots of chronic health issues. As medical and psychological research has shown repeatedly, the body and mind are at work together and can cause chronic health issues. As health-care providers, it is our view that there are body and mind aspects to every physical issue. In the chapters that follow, we offer the three elements of BAM Therapy. The therapy for back issues and their symptoms include the following:

- Physical exercises and treatments

- Spiritual mind treatments

- Affirmations to help the mind and body reconnect with positive healing

The BAM Therapy treatment offers you the opportunity to realize a truth from the Science of Mind perspective: change your thinking, and you change your experience.

PART 2

Getting Started

CHAPTER 3

Be Proactive, Not Reactive

I am the master of my fate. I am the captain of my soul.
-WILLIAM ERNEST HENLEY

When we face an injury, illness, or disease, our natural instinct is to be reactive to the ailment. However, when we are proactive, we take responsibility for our health and wellness on every level.

We can do all the praying, treatments, or affirmations we want, but until we "treat and get off our feet," we are only doing part of the work of healing our ailments. Disease and illness start in the mind and are influenced by our beliefs, our conditioning, and our past. The treatments and affirmations we present here deal with the inner life, the soul. Only our consciousness—our inner being—knows the real source of what ails us. Our consciousness has the ability to heal by replacing old negativity with what we desire to experience.

It is the power within that we go to, and sometimes that inner power knows more than our conscious mind. Going within to find the power to heal often results in better healing than relying on the physical or outward parts of life alone. More and more studies of pain and healing are showing that the inner life is often underdeveloped. If your back is in pain, go within to ask your highest source, your subconscious mind, what is causing the outward symptom. Your innermost self knows the answer. This means that you must prepare to do the work that is necessary to alleviate the symptoms. It is helpful at this point to see a practitioner or doctor who understands the dynamic between the body and the mind and treats the cause of the problem rather than just its symptoms.

Being proactive means taking responsibly for our actions and being willing to change whatever we need to change to move forward in life. One of the most powerful descriptions of being proactive comes from psychologist and neurologist Viktor Frankl, a survivor of the Nazi death camps. Frankl lost all of his family except his sister in the concentration camps. In his classic work *Man's Search for Meaning*, he writes, "Between stimulus and response there is a space. In that space is our power to choose our response." In the concentration camp, Frankl seemingly had no choice in anything. He came to realize that there was space between stimulus and response and that in the space was choice. Frankl chose hope. He chose not to hate his captors. He chose to help his fellow prisoners in any way possible. He chose to find meaning in his suffering.

This is an extreme example of being proactive, yet it exposes a universal truth about human nature and human agency. We do hold the power to take control of our lives— by not letting circumstances and conditions control us and by being proactive rather than reactive. When reactive people experience ailments, their response is to let the pain control them. Reactive people don't act; rather, they are acted upon. A proactive person finds ways to take action in any situation or circumstance. This proactive position is incredibly empowering.

Being Aware of Your Body

Take ten minutes to practice being aware of your body; go within and see what comes up for you physically or emotionally. Start by focusing on your breath for at least one minute. Inhale through the nose and exhale through the mouth as slowly and deeply as you can. As you breathe, focus in turn on your feet, calves, knees, thighs, pelvis, back, neck, and head. Become aware of the sensations in each area without judgment. Just note what you are sensing.

When you focus on your back region, become aware of your straight back. The most common place to hold fear and pain is the neck, mid-back, and lower back regions. This is because the spine represents our life force. It is our backbone—literally and figuratively. When we feel afraid, our backbone can collapse if not taken care of through spiritual thinking and physical movement.

Whatever is going on, we can rely on our life force for one of two things. We can either allow it to boost us up through proper thinking, spiritual mind treatment, affirmations, and physical corrective exercise, or we can ignore it and continue to complain about the condition, doing nothing that may help the problem. In other words, we can be either proactive or reactive. Whether you are dealing with a physical ailment or an emotional one, any ailment will be stuck and cause havoc until you do something proactive.

We must be diligent in checking out what is going on with our minds and bodies. They reflect our relationships and how we maneuver through life, work, and play. For me (Risa), the best time to check in with myself is in the morning, when it is quiet, before I start my day. Checking in with myself first thing in the morning puts me in a positive state of mind. Beginning the day by doing a spiritual treatment sets me in the right emotional and spiritual space for taking on whatever the day brings my way. Moving my body in the correct way also prepares me for whatever the day has in store, and I am confident I can remain proactive no matter what happens.

Usually, when we project our intention in a positive and aligned way, our day goes better because we attract what we put out. Do negative things happen? Of course, they do. But keeping our minds and bodies aligned and looking toward the positive reinforces to the universe that being proactive is the best way to live in the present moment.

Other practices can be adopted to help you take a proactive approach, such as keeping a diary of your ailments and symptoms, noting when they occur over a two-week period, and creating a space at home where you can be alone, such as a room where no one can bother you. Settle in, light a candle or incense, create a small altar with meaningful objects, and create your BAM space.

CHAPTER 4
Tell Me Where It Hurts

New beginnings are often disguised as painful endings.
-LAO TZU

We have all lived in our bodies since birth, and most people think they know their bodies. However, in our culture of excessive stimulation, excessive scheduling, and excessive everything, most people are still strangers to their own bodies. As a result, they are unaware of the potential source of their pain or ailment. We begin this chapter by addressing that problem.

There are many simple body awareness practices you can do to become more aware of your body. Before you start an awareness practice, turn off your phone, lock the door, and create a quiet, contemplative setting.

Meditate: Meditate for a few minutes on a short affirmation. Here is an example: "There is that within me that is whole, perfect, and complete, that which knows the truth. I welcome the day with joy and love. I have a joyous expectation of good for this day. I have joy within, and I attract joy to me."

Stretch: We recommend that you begin and end each day with ten to fifteen minutes of simple stretching exercises. As you stretch, focus on the parts of your body that are stretching. Is it a good stretch with a good sense of exertion, or is it more painful than you think it should be? Adjust accordingly and see how the stretching of your body improves over the next few weeks.

Center: When you center yourself, you connect your mind and body. Locate your center. It can be between the belly button and pubic bone or an inch below the belly button. Visualize moving and stretching from your center as you raise your arms up. Imagine your arms being attached to your center. (See chapter 6 for more on finding your center.)

Body check: Sit upright, your shoulders down and relaxed. Find the center within your body and breathe from that center for three breaths. Mentally scan your body, starting with your head. Is your head tilted? Is one shoulder higher? Are you tight in the shoulder blades? Are your side muscles tight? Is there any pain? Is there tension in any part of your body? Where you feel tension, have your mind say, "Let go," to that part of the body.

Identifying Pain

Let's look at how you can identify chronic pain, day to day, by expanding on the above body awareness work you will do on a daily basis. After your daily check-in exercises of stretching, centering, and walking, step into your BAM space for five minutes to identify any symptoms resulting from daily life and how you are reacting to them.

Breathe. Think about your daily life and how you react to what life brings you. Use the BAM Body Map (see figure 4.1) to better understand your body symptoms and how they might impact your emotional being. The BAM Body Map shows the six zones of the back and where emotional stress typically manifests.

HUMAN VERTEBRAL COLUMN

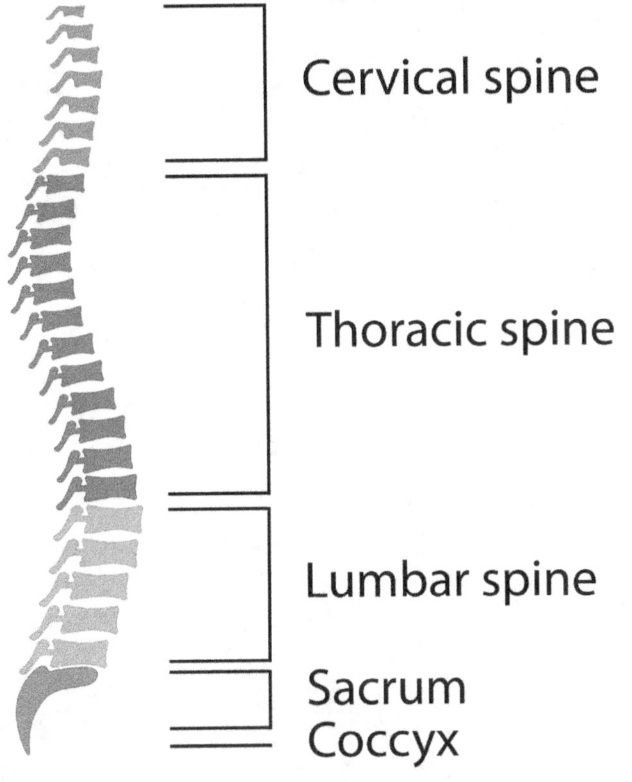

FIGURE 4.1

Please note that as a generalization, gender and age are factors in your health. Generally speaking, women tend to be thinkers and more emotionally developed, while men are more reticent to talk about issues and tend to exert more physical effort. Consequently, women tend to have headaches and neck and shoulder ailments, while men tend to have stomach and lower back issues.

CHAPTER 5
Breath, Breathing, and the Back

To breathe properly is to live properly
-Robin Sharma

As we write this, we are in the middle of a pandemic, the likes of which the world has not experienced in more than a century. The COVID-19 pandemic has not only slowed down our lives and activities, but it has also provided a lesson of utmost importance: breathe slowly, deeply, and mindfully. Like the back, the breath is what gives us support and the ability to live our lives.

The coronavirus seems to attack the respiratory system the hardest. Those with compromised respiratory systems, along with senior citizens, appear to be the most vulnerable to the virus. Now is the time to develop and control our breathing. It is our life force. We have very little control over much of our lives, but we do have complete control of how we breathe.

In my Pilates teaching, I have always stressed the importance of breath. It is one of the six main components of movement that define Pilates. Joe Pilates said, "Breathing is the first act of life and the last. Our very life depends on it. It is tragically deplorable to contemplate the millions who have never mastered the art of correct breathing."

I (Risa) have been using deep breathing in my practice for forty-some years. As I have gone deeper into meditation, I have experienced more profoundly the coordination of mind, body, and spirit, with breathing being the common denominator. I realized firsthand that most of us don't breathe deeply. Shallow breathing seems to be the norm. I have observed that movement becomes easier and that minds become clearer with correct breathing. Our overall well-being is inextricably entwined with correct breathing.

Breathing Mind Treatment

Close your eyes and go within. Repeat the following as you breathe deeply and rhythmically.

I am one with the infinite One.

I am one with the spirit, the universal god.

I breathe in the spirit of life, and I am a living soul.

I am whole, perfect, and complete.

All sense of restriction, fear, and anxiety of any kind is released through the power of this treatment.

Nothing can negate this life force within me.

I am a magnet for good. I release all fear, all judgment, and all self-blame.

I am responsible for myself, and I see and accept only good, love, and support.

I am grateful for this awareness, and I joyously release this word out into the universe, knowing it returns to me abundantly.

Breathing exercise

Sit in a chair, with your back straight and your feet on the floor. Place your hands on your lap or across your heart.

Take a deep breath, count to eight, hold for four counts, then exhale through your mouth for a count of eight.

Focus on your breathing and breathing alone. If other thoughts come up, just let them pass without judgment and move on to the next breath. Repeat this five times.

If your mind wanders, bring it back to your breathing.

After a few minutes of this deep breathing, say this to yourself: "I love life. I am safe. I breathe in the breath of God, and I am a living soul. I am one with all living things."

These affirmations, along with silent deep breathing, will increase your endorphins and negate fear.

Staying focused on life-affirming thoughts helps us keep our minds and hearts in the right place to create good in our lives and the lives of others.

BAM Therapy for Common Ailments

CHAPTER 6
Finding Your Center

You have to be able to center yourself, to let all of your emotions go. Don't ever forget that you play with your soul as well as your body.
-KAREEM ABDUL-JABBAR

Finding your center is like building a house. You first need a solid foundation to hold up the house. Similarly, without a healthy trunk, a tree cannot sustain its own branches, leaves, or fruit. The body is the same, but for human beings, the foundation consists of spiritual or mental stability from which the physical body flows.

We often associate the word *exercise* with drudgery, something to put off until tomorrow, next week, or next year. The word *movement* conveys joy and freedom, something we all like to experience. We want you to think of this program for better health as a series of movements and not a series of exercises. The movements you are about to learn are part of Risa's Sheppard Method of movements, which is rooted in her Pilates training. They are not fast, jerky, or difficult movements but free-flowing, graceful motions that show results without pain or strain.

Over one hundred years ago, Joe Pilates said, "You are as young as your spine is flexible." That means that as we grow older, neglecting correct posture and spinal articulation will lead to a compressed spine, causing everything from spinal stenosis to a herniated disc and a lot of pain. Pilates instructor Aliyah Hatcher describes spinal articulation as "the ability to move the bones of your spine, or your vertebrae, in segments, piece by piece, sequentially."[9]

Think of your spine like a string of pearls. The vertebrae are like individual pearls held together with strings of equal length in between each one, holding them in alignment with the natural curvature of the back. It helps to number the vertebra or pearls so you can imagine the string lengthening as your hold your back straight, feeling the pearls separate (see the diagram of the spine on p.33). Imagine the spine extending beyond the crown of your head and growing higher and higher.

Using these visualizations of spine lengthening in the following exercises will help your muscles loosen around the spine, creating more flexibility while strengthening the entire back and abdominals to create a longer, more flexible body and mind.

How to Find Your Center

The movements to follow are designed to strengthen and affirm the most important part of the body: its center. By developing the center, you will create firmer and flatter abdominals, a stronger lower back, better posture, and a trimmer waist. The center provides the strength and control

---

9   Cited in Rachel Lapidos, "6 Spinal Articulation Pilates Exercises to Do For a Healthy, Mobil Back," Well + Good, https://www.wellandgood. com/spinal-articulation/.

necessary to perform all exercise movements and better prepares your body for other sports and activities.

The main emphasis on developing your center is to create abdominals that are flat and not rounded. Most people do abdominals incorrectly by sticking their stomachs out during the exercise. In order to get the most benefit, do each movement slowly, concentrating on holding the stomach muscles firm and flat toward the spine. This takes a certain amount of concentration at first, but it will soon become a habit. And you will find that the results are phenomenal.

FINDING YOUR CENTER EXERCISE

Developing a strong, firm center begins with proper body alignment. The first exercise is the essential starting point for your daily movements. Stand sideways in front of a full-length mirror with your legs spread slightly apart. Notice how you are standing. Is your stomach protruding? Is your back swayed? Are your shoulders hunched?

Begin by gently squeezing your buttocks and aiming your tailbone toward the floor. Next, lift your rib cage and elongate your waist. I call this declumping. (Most of us tend to clump in the midsection.) Relax and slightly pull back the shoulders. Place your right hand on the lower abdominals and your left hand on

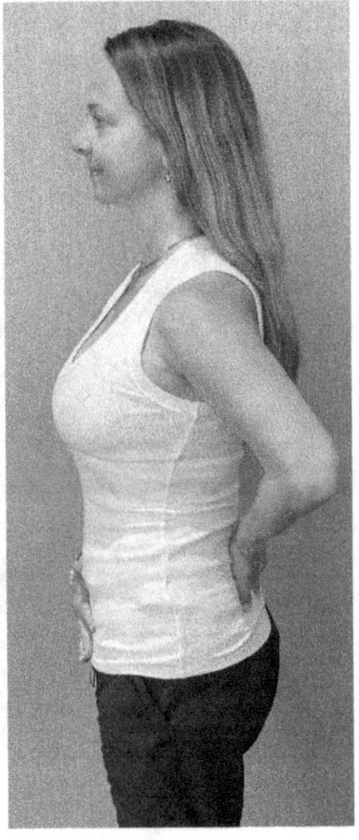

FIGURE 6.1

the lower back. (See figure 6.1.) The area you are holding is your center.

Now place the index fingers of both hands on your hips, pointing toward your insides. Imagine a laser beam running through your body between your fingers. You are pointing to your center. (See figure 6.2.)

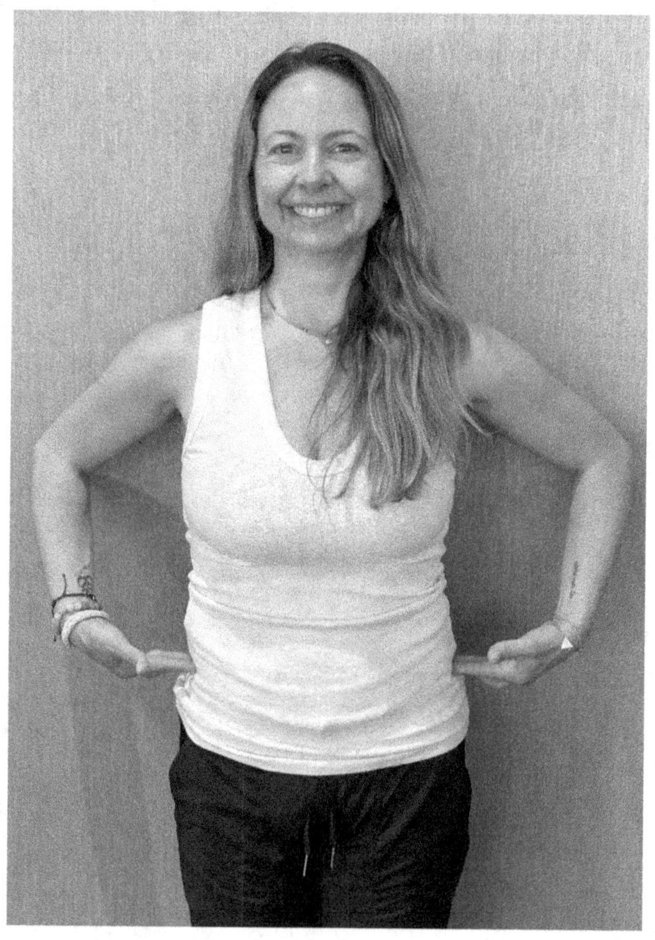

FIGURE 6.2

Breathing from your center. Now that you have found your center, you will begin some deep breathing. Deep breathing is the aerobic conditioning in BAM Therapy. We often take this aerobic breathing exercise for granted, not realizing how important it is.

Proper breathing is an essential part of doing any movement correctly and efficiently. When doing these movements, always breathe deeply and slowly, inhaling through the nose and exhaling through the mouth. Never hold your breath during any movement.

Now begin. As you hold in your center (see figure 6.1), inhale through your nose as you extend your arms overhead. Exhale through your mouth as you slowly lower your arms. Repeat three times.

CHAPTER 7

The Cranial Region

There is a wisdom of the head, and a wisdom of the heart.
-Charles Dickens

The cranial region is the upper part of the head and includes where the brain resides. The cranial region represents the mind in both its positive appreciation of the beauty of the world and its confusion with the world around and within us. Cranial ailments manifest in the body as migraines, dizziness, fatigue, and colds. As physical and metaphysical healers, we can heal these symptoms with mental treatment and corrective exercise using Pilates, Sheppard Method Pilates principles, and chiropractic treatments.

Symptoms

Symptoms from cranial stress usually manifest as the following ailments:

- Migraines and headaches
- Disturbed sleep cycles and insomnia
- Neck pain
- Temporomandibular joint dysfunction or TMJ

- Trauma, including trauma from whiplash
- Mood disorders
- Sinus infections
- Irritable bowel syndrome

Probable Causes

When objectively looking at the probable causes of cranial troubles, you must begin by looking at what is taking place in your life that is causing confusion. What emotions are you experiencing that may trigger these symptoms? Perhaps you do not know where you stand in your primary relationship, with family, or at work. Is there duality in your thinking, a simultaneous holding of two separate ideas that contradict each other? For example, you may work with someone you don't like, so you have to push down your emotions to do your work. This withholding of emotion can cause cranial ailments. Do you hold confusing thoughts about a specific subject, wondering, *Should I? Shouldn't I?* This can lead to overload within the mind, and a roaring headache or dizziness may occur because your thoughts are not clear. We are usually distraught over such contradictions.

The goal is to stop what you are thinking, get still, and go within using a spiritual mind treatment.

Case Study: John

John had been suffering from headaches since he returned from a military tour of duty to Afghanistan. A strong young man, he had done his tour and never had any complaints. Once he came home to his wife and baby boy, John awakened each day with a stiff neck and a pounding head. He took aspirin to reduce the pain, but the symptoms soon returned. He had visited his doctor, but they could not determine what was causing the headaches.

John was referred to me (David). After hearing of John's recent past overseas, I began asking questions about what was going on now with his new "old" life and what that was like for him.

"To be honest," John explained, "having the responsibility of a wife and newborn is scarier to me than being at war. I'm having a hard time adjusting to making decisions for my son's future and being a good husband to Naomi, my wife."

I knew that this was the case for BAM Therapy. Risa and I talked more with John about his fears and feelings. We understood that a common mental equivalent for head and neck pain is often self-criticism and fear. John criticized himself for not being able to save his friend in Afghanistan. He felt that he was not a good soldier and therefore could not possibly be a good husband and father. This self-criticism was robbing him of enjoyment in his life at home and eventually developed into a false sense of responsibility; he had put the whole ordeal of Afghanistan on his shoulders. The tighter his shoulders became, the worse the headaches were. Risa and I knew what the next step should be: rid John of his false sense of responsibility and self-criticism.

After a month of BAM Therapy, which included exercises for the neck and shoulders, mind treatment, and affirmations, John's headaches were gone. Today he is free of headaches and pain, and he now enjoys his family and his work as an electrician.

BAM Therapy Routine for the Cranial Region

The following movement will help relieve cranial pain.

SHOULDER MOVEMENT.

1. Lift your shoulders as high as you can. (See figure 7.1.)
2. Drop your shoulders as if someone is pressing them down. Feel the shoulders relax. (See figure 7.2.)
3. Repeat three times.

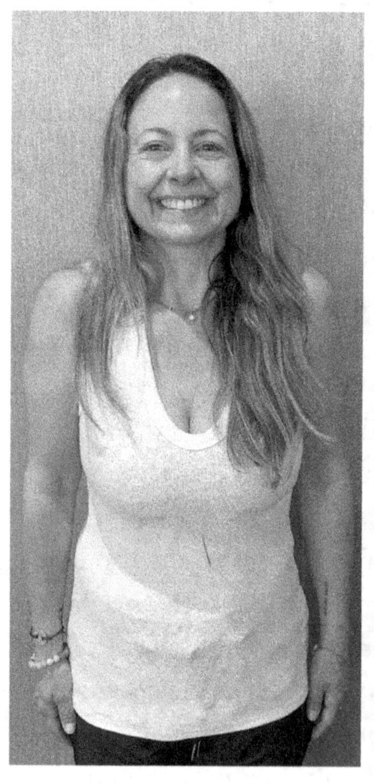

FIGURE 7.1

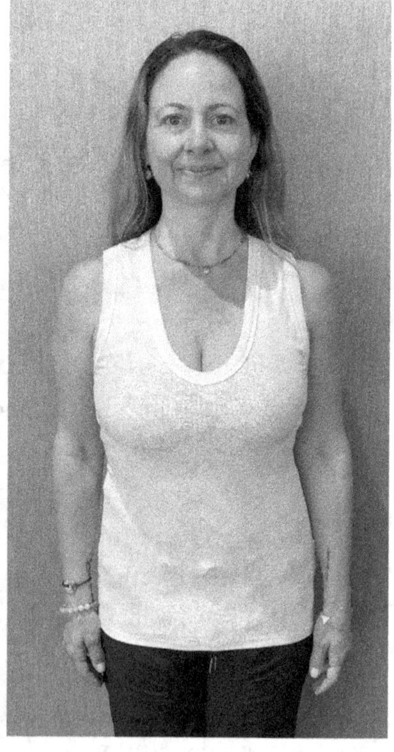

FIGURE 7.2

Spiritual Mind Treatment

There is one idea, one power, one perfect idea in the mind of the spirit.

There is no contradiction, no separation, and no confusion, only oneness and right action.

Anything contrary to the perfect idea of the spirit is null and void through the power of this treatment.

I am clear knowing, clear thinking, and clear understanding.

Anything in my subconscious that does not believe in the wholeness of the universe is made null and void by the power of this word.

My word has power. I dissolve any thoughts of lack, loss, or limitation of any kind. I am all-knowing, all-powerful, whole, and complete.

And so it is.

Affirmation

"I am one mind, one power, and one life. I know what to do and do it with confidence."

CHAPTER 8

The Cervical Region

Watch the turtle. He only moves forward
by sticking his neck out.
-Louis V. Gerstner, Jr.

The cervical region starts at the root of the brain stem and continues to the base of the neck. It controls the eyes, ears, nose, and sinuses. Those who complain of headaches, sinus ailments, or dizziness often have their cervical spine out of alignment, and it needs to be realigned. As this part of the spine controls the movement of the head itself, the cervical region metaphysically represents the ability to be flexible in our views and thinking, look at all parts of a situation, and be open to new ways of perceiving a problem.

Symptoms

Symptoms of cervical problems usually manifest as the following ailments:

- Stiff neck
- Pain in upper arms or shoulders
- Tendonitis
- Bursitis

- Herniated disc
- Numbing through the arms and fingers

Probable Causes

One of the most common causes of cervical problems is repressed anger. Such anger, whether stemming from childhood or from a present condition, can aggravate the cervical area, stopping proper blood flow and causing confusion. Look at where you are angry, either now or in your past. Let go of the anger and the frustration at not having things the way you want them. Look around and find the beauty that is all around you.

The neck and shoulder regions allow us to turn our sight and mind to whatever is around us at any given time. It makes sense that the cervical spine represents the ability to see all sides of a situation, focus our attention on whatever is happening around us, and be open and receptive to what we see. Most people are not willing to see all sides of a situation before making a judgment or decision. In fact, many of us are unaware of or unwilling to give up our view of a situation and consider other possibilities. That inflexibility in life corresponds to pain and inflexibility in the neck and shoulders.

Look at your life as it is right now. Is there something specific you are not looking at? Something too hurtful? Is there anger associated with something you are avoiding? Is there someone that you cannot forgive? Are you refusing to understand another's point of view? It doesn't matter if you can identify the actual situation or idea; it may be so buried within that you cannot understand it, accept it, or recognize it. That's okay. Your subconscious mind knows and remembers everything.

Case Study 1: James

James came to my chiropractic office with severe neck pain. He was unable to turn his head, and he told me he had never had pain like this before. After doing a complete consultation and exam plus a full set of x-rays, I noted that James's neck region was within normal limits. His neck pain seemed to lie deeper than what could be discerned through a careful exam of his body.

I asked James what was going on with him emotionally and if there were life issues causing him stress. He replied, "No, nothing."

Later that day, I called him to check up on how he was feeling. He said he had been thinking about what I asked him, about what was going on with him emotionally. He then told me that the night before he came for treatment, he and his wife had told their five-year-old daughter that they were getting divorced. He asked me, "Do you think that has something to do with this physical pain?" I said, "Absolutely."

We gave him a treatment to do daily. We suggested breathing exercises combined with a spiritual mind treatment to release the pain and irritation and allow him to feel free once again.

Each morning on awakening, James closed his eyes and practiced the BAM Therapy regimen we prescribed. The breathing exercise provided him with deep relaxation as well as the curative value of positive autosuggestion (see chapter 5). As he inhaled, he imagined energy coming into his cervical spine. As he exhaled, he imagined the energy being directed into the affected body point, driving out the pain and healing it. Once he finished the breathing exercise, he felt completely relaxed and at peace.

With his eyes still closed, he then spoke the following spiritual mind treatment out loud:

I am the spirit. The spirit within me is perfect, whole, and complete.

There is one divine life in the universe, and that life is alive in me right here and right now.

All sense of lack, loss, or limitation is dissolved from my consciousness.

There is only light, love, and joy emanating from within me and without me.

Anything in me that finds it hard to see all sides of every situation or any part of me that has been harboring fear or resentment is completely liberated through the power of this word.

We also suggested this affirmation: "I release all fear, and I embrace love." James used this short and powerful affirmation throughout the day in moments when he felt alone and experienced fear.

To aid in his physical healing and strengthen his body, we gave James several BAM Therapy exercises to do following the breathing exercise and spiritual mind treatment. The exercises are detailed following case study 2.

First, James does the Finding Your Center exercise (see chapter 6). It was important for him to experience being strong emotionally and understand that he can provide this feeling for himself and overcome his fears. It was equally important for him to experience the physical sensation of having a strong body, as this could work the other way around and help him feel stronger emotionally. The two aspects—physical and emotional—work together to support each other, and, when used in unison, speed up the healing process.

As he did the "finding your center" exercise, he also spoke the following affirmation: "I am centered, calm, and balanced."

Next, James did neck exercises. These exercises stretched and loosened his cervical spine muscles, helping the muscles support the spine and reduce inflammation (and fear).

He then spoke this affirmation: "I am clear in my communication."

By following these exercises, James has strengthened his neck and improved his posture. He starts each day with BAM Therapy, finding his center, doing the neck exercises, and speaking the affirmations. He has now moved to a new house and has joint custody of his daughter. He is in a new relationship and is very happy. He would like his ex-wife to start the BAM Therapy too as it helped him so much to get through this hard time.

Case Study 2: Helen

Helen came to me about three years ago. Helen, a fifty-five-year-old director of a university hospital, is responsible for the upkeep and health of elderly Alzheimer patients.

At the time she first came to see me, her elderly mother was giving her a lot of grief about family matters. Helen was feeling stuck. She developed a pinched nerve in her neck, making it almost impossible to turn her head in either direction. Her mother was demanding her time, and her patients were demanding her constant attention.

After we chatted for a bit, she admitted that she was feeling frustrated and that no one understood the pressure they were putting on her. She was having difficulty seeing her mother's side of the problem and those of her patients. She was unable to see all sides of these situations.

I thought that the pinched nerve in her neck was the result of seeing only one side of what was going on. She was feeling stuck, believing that there was no way out for anyone and that there was only one way to look at the situation: her way.

We prescribed a spiritual mind treatment to help Helen get unstuck and relieve her neck pain: "There is only one mind, one truth, and one life, and this life is my life. I am perfect, whole, and complete. All thoughts of lack, limitation, or fear are completely absolved by the power of this treatment. All past traumas that have resulted in an inability to see other perspectives are removed from my consciousness now and forever."

Helen is now able to live her life free of constraint, condemnation, and fear. She is able to see all sides of a situation, and she accepts life as it is. Nothing is pinched. Nothing is constrained. She is perfect, her patients are in the right place, and her mother is in the right place. All is well.

We also suggested Helen repeat the following affirmation: "I am flexible in all areas of my life. I accept all situations without judgment. I accept all that life has to offer."

BAM Therapy Routine for the Cervical region

The following movements will help relieve cervical pain.

MOVEMENT 1: NECK AND SHOULDER STRETCH

1. Stand or sit erect, with your spine straight, elongating the spine from your tailbone to above your head. Drop your shoulders away from your ears. Lengthen your neck as you inhale. Drop your chin to your chest in a slow and deliberate manner as you exhale. Hold for five counts and then lift your head up. Repeat three times. (See figures 8.1 and 8.2.)

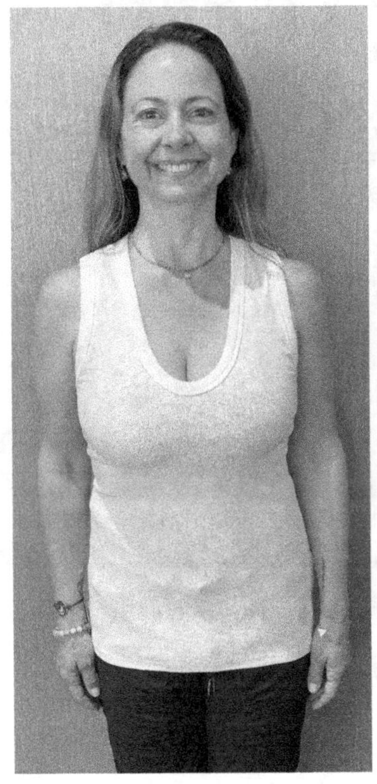

FIGURE 8.1

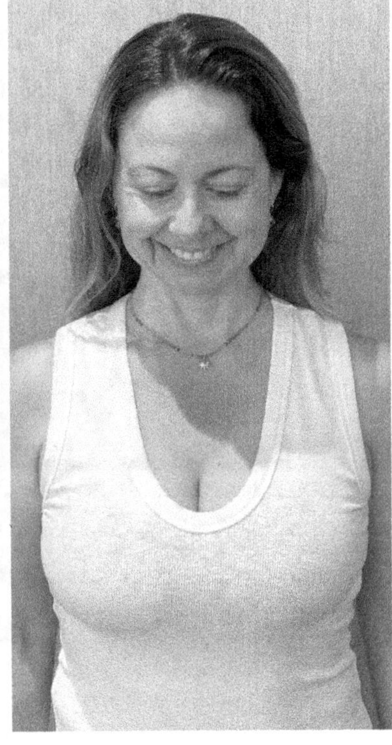

FIGURE 8.2

2. Slowly and deliberately turn your head to the right. As you turn, imagine moving your chin directly over your right shoulder. Hold for five counts. Repeat three to four times. (See figure 8.3.)

3. Slowly and deliberately turn your head to the left. As you turn, imagine moving your chin directly over your left shoulder. Hold for five counts. Repeat three to four times. (See figure 8.4.)

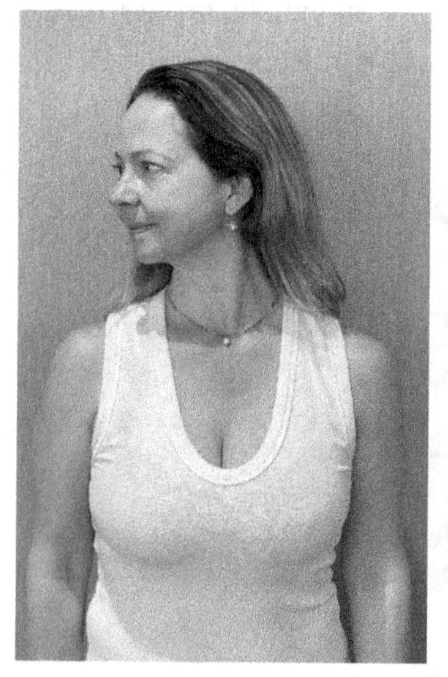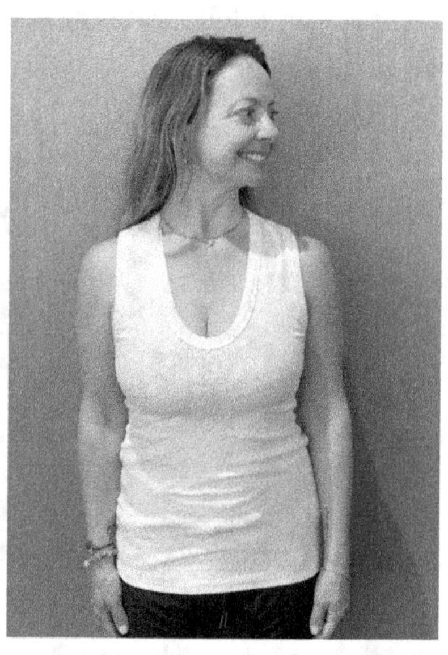

FIGURE 8.3   **FIGURE 8.4**

4. Look forward. Bring your left hand around the top of your head and cover your right ear. Gently press your head toward your left shoulder. Feel the stretch on the right side of the neck. Hold for five seconds. (See figure 8.5.)

5. Look forward. Bring your right hand over your head and cover your left ear. Gently press your head toward your right shoulder. Feel the stretch on the left side of your neck. Hold for five seconds. (See figure 8.6.)

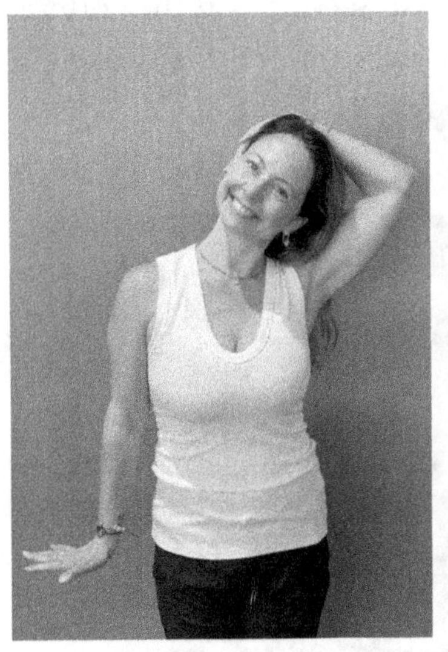

FIGURE 8.5

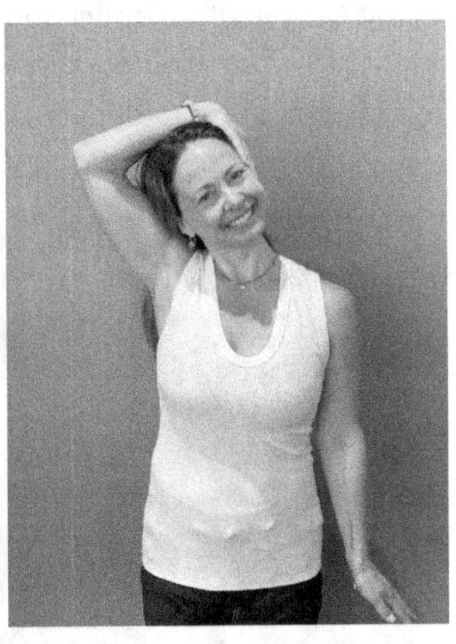

FIGURE 8.6

MOVEMENT 2: CHEST OPENING

You will need a foam roller for this movement.

1. Place the foam roller lengthwise on a yoga mat or towel.
2. Sit on one end of the roller. Lie back so that your head is at the top of the roller and your sacrum is at the bottom.
3. Reach your arms out to the sides and feel the stretching in your chest and upper body. (See figure 8.7.)

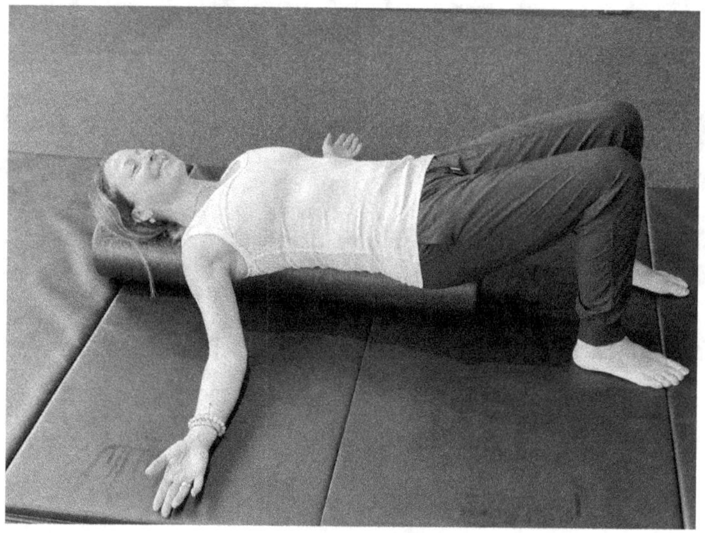

FIGURE 8.7

4. Remain on the foam roller. Bend your knees so that your feet are flat on the floor. Raise your arms together toward the ceiling. (See figure 8.8.)

5. Keeping your arms straight, extend your right arm above your head, parallel to the floor, as you extend your left arm toward your feet. (See figure 8.9.)

6. Alternate your arms up and down ten times. (See figure 8.10.)

Repeat this affirmation after the exercises

"I move through life with ease."

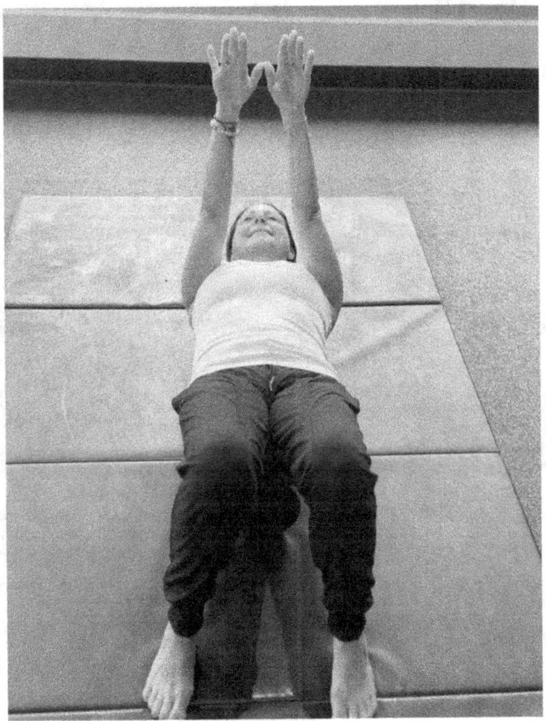

FIGURE 8.8

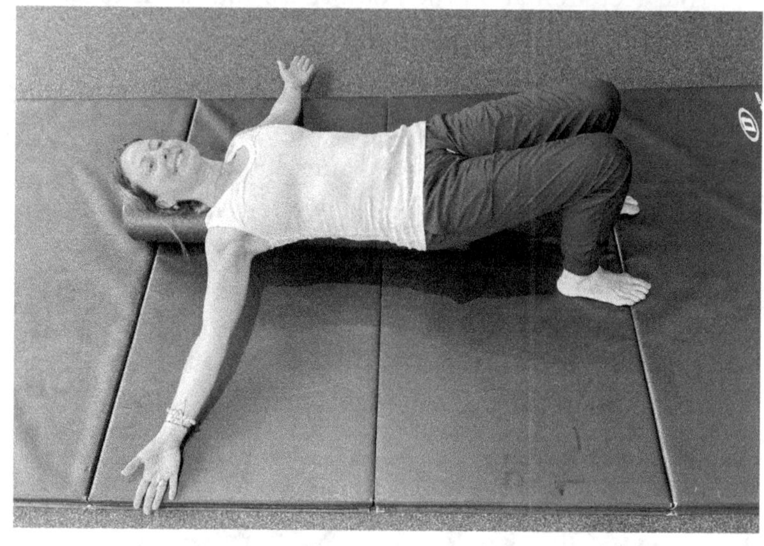

FIGURE 8.9

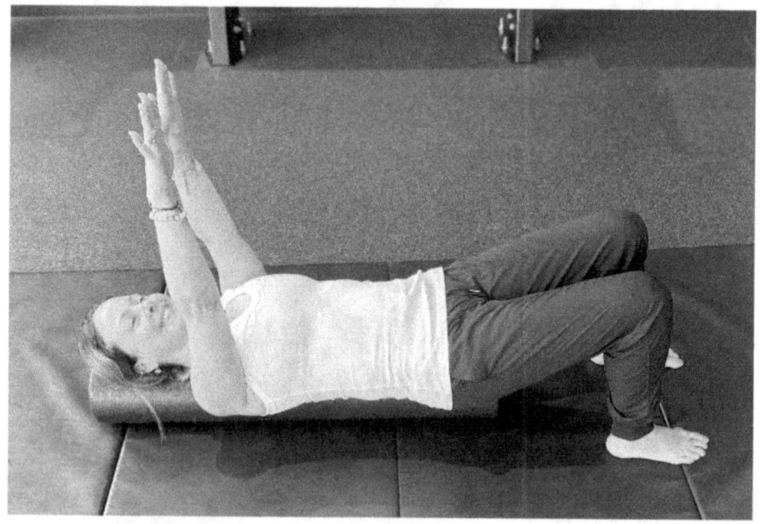

FIGURE 8.10

Spiritual mind treatment

I go within and call on the Infinite Presence that dwells within me.

This Presence is omniscient, omnipresent, and omnipotent.

This Presence within me now dissolves all past limitations, losses, and fear of the unknown.

I am now willing and able to accept all sides of a situation, either in the past or present.

I lovingly release all tension, rigid thinking, and fear that can constrict my body in any way.

I let go. I let God do his perfect work through me and as me.

For God is within me now, has always been within me, and always will be.

And so it is.

Affirmation

"I easily look at all sides of a situation and am flexible and nonjudgmental in my thinking. I am one mind, one power, and one life. I know what to do and do it with confidence. I am flexible in all my ways."

CHAPTER 9
The Thoracic Region

A healthy mind has an easy breath.
-Dr. David Tannenbaum

The thoracic region is the area in the mid back. Although the thoracic spine controls many bodily functions, the most common issues we see here in clients and patients are caused by emotions. This is, after all, the heart region. When we work with clients who have particular thoracic weakness, pain, or tightness, we ask, "Is there anything going on love-wise with you?" This could be romantic or otherwise.

The thoracic region is not as movable as the cervical or lumbar regions, so it can sometimes harbor an emotion for years without you feeling the effects. But years of neglect can take its toll. It is important to always maintain proper support, both physically and emotionally. The spine is our life support in all areas. Keeping it maintained, both physically and emotionally, is of utmost importance.

We find this area of the back interesting and extremely challenging. Unlike the cranial and cervical (head and neck) regions and the lumbar (lower back) region, where most injuries rest, the thoracic region can be the most vulnerable place to store unresolved emotions.

Some practitioners and healers relate the thoracic region to the heart chakra in yoga—the area that represents issues of loss, love, hurt, and pain. When a chiropractic patient comes to me, complaining of a tight thoracic back, one of the first questions I ask is if they have a problem in or with their love life, such as a divorce, a breakup, or even death. It doesn't have to be a romantic issue, though.

Symptoms

Symptoms in the thoracic region usually manifest as the following ailments:

- Stiffness

- Digestive problems

- Asthma

- Muscle weakness

- Muscle spasms

- Stooped posture

- Thoracic nerve pain, which can manifest in symptoms such as numbness or burning pain

Probable Causes

The Thoracic Spine is the middle section of your back. It starts at the base of your neck and ends at the bottom of your ribs. It is especially ridge and stable, unlike the cervical and lumbar spine.

The Thoracic spine area corresponds to the "heart Chakra." It is known to represent and manifest as anything to do with affairs of "the heart." It does not mean just romance, it includes all emotional relationships and feelings. The thoracic rigidity can be a barrier to feelings of the heart.

Let's take my client Anne. Age 54, Anne is a recovering anorexic and alcoholic. Her body was as stiff as a board. She complained of pain and stiffness in her thoracic, or middle spine as she called it. After some time of helping her physically, I felt comfortable enough to ask her if she had any feelings of heartbreak she was harboring. She turned to me and started weeping that her Mother had never loved her, and her mother made a point of telling Anne often of this fact.

She had an older sibling that she felt her Mother always loved so much more.

And all this was over 50 years ago! You can imagine what the use of alcohol plus feelings of loss of love was doing to her body. All the exercise in the world would not soften her heart and the feelings around it.

It took a while, but with some Mind treatment and the simple affirmation "I am love" Anne has increased the mobility in her spine that had been locked for so long. When feelings of not being loved now arise, she can immediately turn within, claim the love that is within her, and move her spine in ways that relieve pain, as her heart and mind accept her new feelings of love and acceptance.

Case Study 1: Robert

Robert came to the office with trouble taking a deep breath. He was experiencing severe chest pains beyond anything he had felt before. After doing a full consultation, exams, and a full set of x-rays, his physical body seemed within normal limits. Robert also went to his general medical practitioner and had a full medical workup and exam, and everything appeared normal.

I asked him what was going on emotionally. He told me he had recently switched careers and was having a lot of anxiety related to the pandemic and financial responsibilities to support his family. The thoracic area of the spine is correlated to the heart, chest, and abdominal areas, so the fear of failing at his new position, coupled with feeling overwhelmed at the possibility of the loss of love and respect from his family and friends, was likely contributing to his symptoms.

We gave him a BAM Therapy treatment to do daily. We suggested breathing exercises combined with a spiritual mind treatment to release the pain and irritation and allow him to feel free once again.

Each morning on awakening, Robert closed his eyes and practiced his BAM Therapy treatment. The breathing exercises provided him with deep relaxation as well as the ability to face the day without fear.

As he inhaled, he imagined energy coming into his entire body. As he exhaled, he imagined in his mind's eye the energy being directed into the affected point, driving out the pain and healing it. Once he finished the breathing, he felt completely relaxed and at peace.

Then, with his eyes still closed, he spoke the following spiritual mind treatment out loud: "I accept life. I take it in easily, and my heart forgives and releases. It is safe to love myself. I claim my own power. I lovingly create my own reality. I open myself to love and joy."

To aid in Robert's physical healing and strengthen his body, we gave him several BAM Therapy exercises to do following his breathing and spiritual mind treatment.

First, he did the Finding Your Center exercise (see chapter 6). As he did the exercise, he spoke the following affirmation: "I am open and receptive to all good. The universe loves and supports me."

Next, he did the BAM Therapy routine for thoracic exercises (see the pages following). These exercises stretch and loosen the thoracic spine muscles, helping the muscles support the spine and reduce inflammation. To release anxiety and fear of the future, Robert recites this affirmation out loud: "I choose to circulate the joys of life."

Robert now starts each day with the BAM thoracic exercises and affirmations. The exercises have strengthened his thoracic spine and improved his posture. He has now started his new career and has been very successful, and he has surrendered his good to the universe as he opens his heart to the unknown.

Case Study 2: Lila

Lila is a sixty-year-old occupational therapist who has struggled with anorexia for most of her adult life. She complained of living with spasms around her thoracic back for years. When I asked if she had any love issues that she was dealing with, she started crying and said, "My mother never loved me. She never even told me she cared, and she said that she in fact favored my older sister. She told me she always resented my coming along. I have lived with that my whole life."

We prescribed the BAM Therapy routine for the thoracic region for Lila and gave her a spiritual mind treatment. After receiving the spiritual mind treatment, Lila felt more relaxed, but the work was just beginning. We gave her this affirmation to repeat daily, if not hourly: "I am loved unconditionally." She also repeated the spiritual mind treatment at the end of this chapter.

With proper treatment through movement, spiritual mind treatment, and affirmations, Lila reduced and eventually eliminated the spasms in her thoracic back.

As Lila's story shows, nothing is too large for our individual minds and spiritual connections to heal.

Lila also repeats this affirmation after her morning therapy: "I am love, expressing love in all that I do and say."

BAM Therapy Routine for the Thoracic Region

The following movements will help relieve thoracic pain.

MOVEMENT 1: BACK STRETCH

1. Interlock your fingers in front of you, palms pointing away. Hollow out your abdominals, and round your back. (See figure 9.1.)
2. Engage your buttocks, and stretch out your arms, keeping your fingers interlocked. Feel the middle of your back stretch wide open. Repeat three times. (See figure 9.2.)

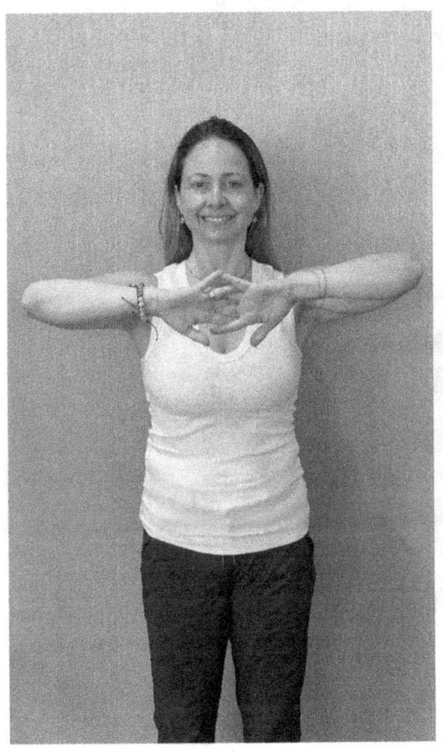

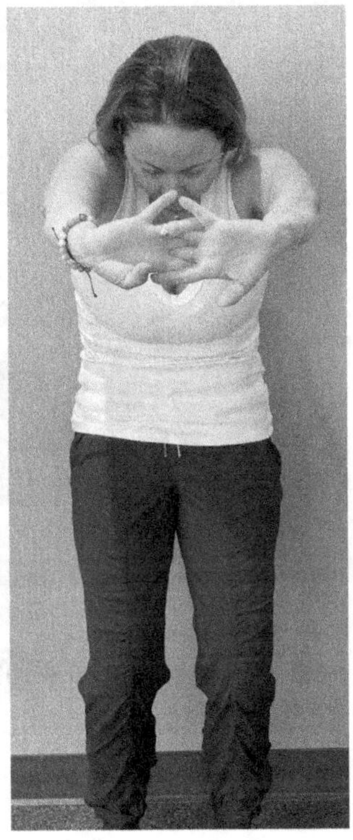

FIGURE 9.1   FIGURE 9.2

3. Keeping your hip bones pointed straight ahead and fingers interlocked, hollow in your abdominals, and round your back. Keeping your hip bones pointed forward, rotate your arms and torso to the right as far as you can reach. Then turn to the left and stretch as far as you can. Feel the stretch in your middle back as you slowly rotate side to side. (See figures 9.3 and 9.4.)

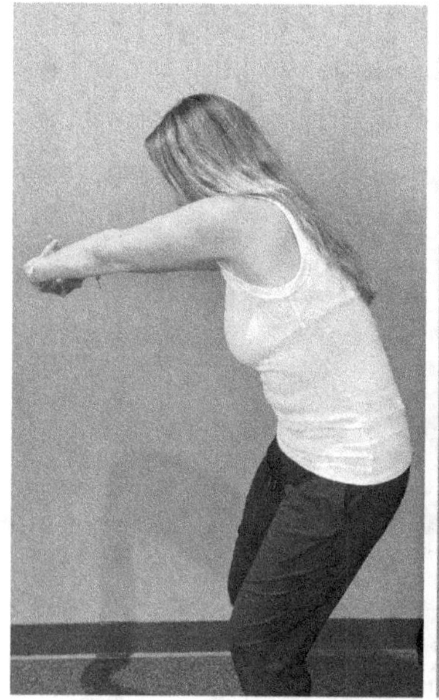

FIGURE 9.3

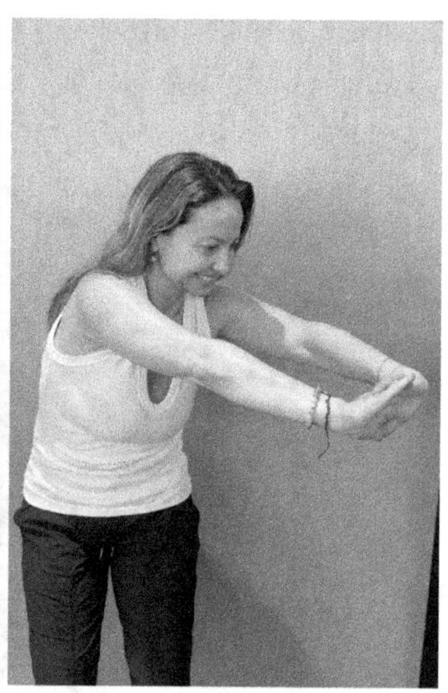

FIGURE 9.4

Repeat this affirmation

"My heart forgives and releases the past. I let life flow through me. All is well."

MOVEMENT 2: CAT-COW

Come to all fours, in a tabletop position, with your arms under your shoulders and your knees under your hips. (See figure 9.5.)

1. Contract your abdominals and round your back like a cat. Tuck your tailbone, pelvis, and cervical spine under. (See figure 9.6.)

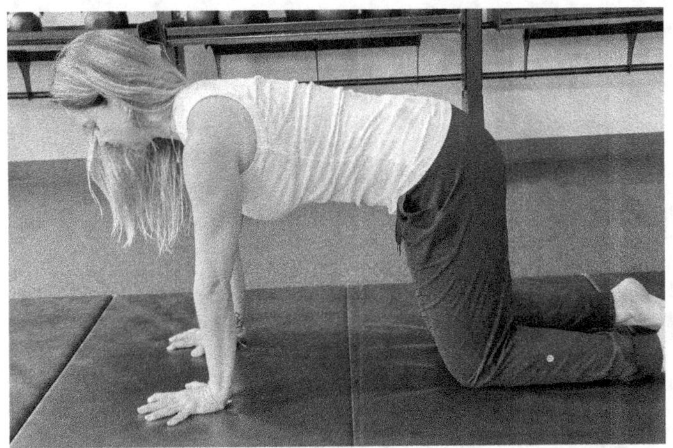

FIGURE 9.5

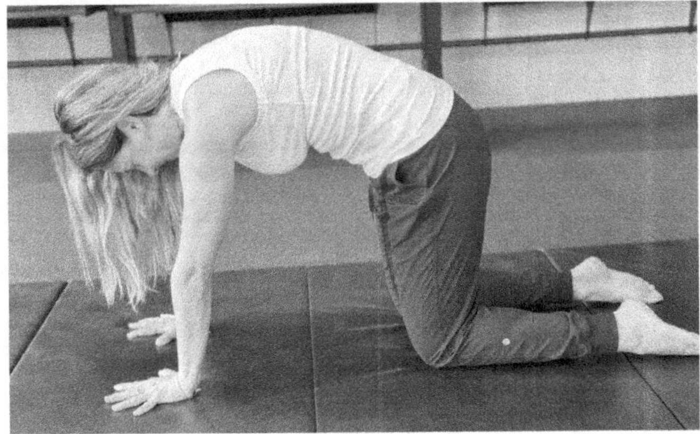

FIGURE 9.6

2. Move through the tabletop position again, slowly and deliberately straightening and elongating your head and spine, making a straight line from the top of your head to your tailbone. Then arch your thoracic back toward the floor while still holding in the abdominals. (See figure 9.7.)

3. Repeat three to five times.

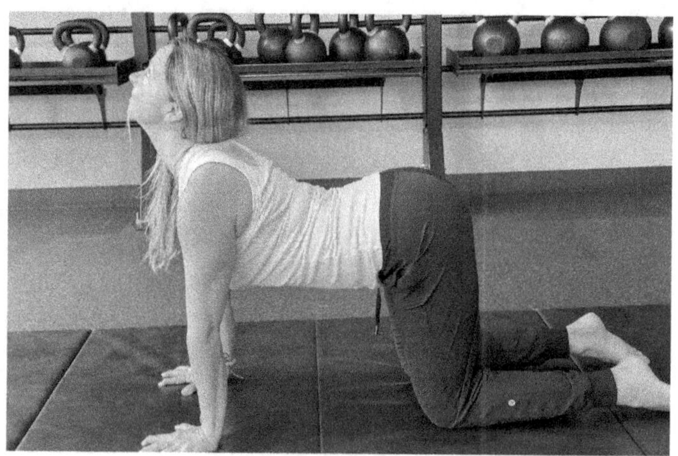

FIGURE 9.7

Repeat this affirmation

"I am open and receptive to all good."

MOVEMENT 3: SPINE ROTATION

1. Sit erect on the floor with your back straight. (You may sit against a wall if you wish.)

2. Keeping your right leg straight, bend your left knee and cross your left foot over your right leg, placing your foot flat on the floor. Place your right hand on your left knee. (See figure 9.8.)

3. Pull into your chest as you lift and twist toward the left as if you are looking behind you. Hold for four counts.

4. Gently come back to the center and repeat on the other side. Stretch your left leg out, bend your right knee over your left leg, and twist toward the right.

5. Each time, feel as though your spine is growing out from above your head.

6. Repeat on each side three to four times.

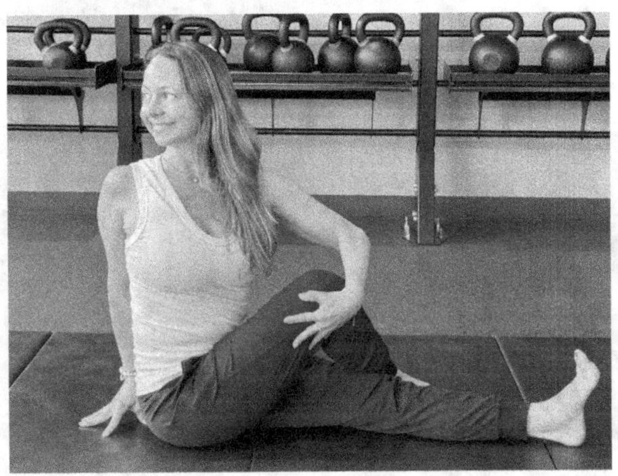

FIGURE 9.8

Repeat this affirmation

"I am willing to move forward in life."

MOVEMENT 4: THORACIC AND LUMBAR SPINE STRETCH

1. Lie supine on a mat, knees bent, feet flat on the floor. Feel your spine pressed against the mat. (See figure 9.9.)
2. Bring your right foot to the outside of your left knee. (See figure 9.10.)

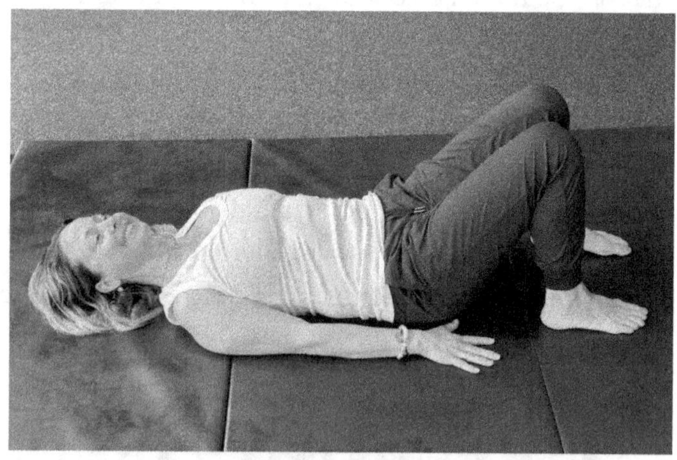

FIGURE 9.9

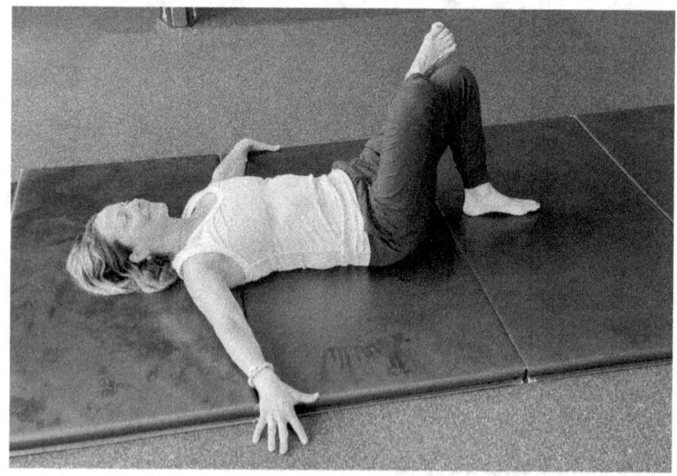

FIGURE 9.10

3. Keeping both shoulders on the floor, gently allow your right foot to lower your left knee toward the right, bringing it as close to the floor as you can take it without lifting your shoulders. Turn your head to the left, feeling the twist in the torso. (See figure 9.11.) Be sure to maintain separation between the bottom of your rib cage and the tip of your hip bone.

4. Hold the stretch for eight to ten counts.

5. Repeat in the opposite direction, placing your left foot over your right knee, and so on. Turn your head to the right.

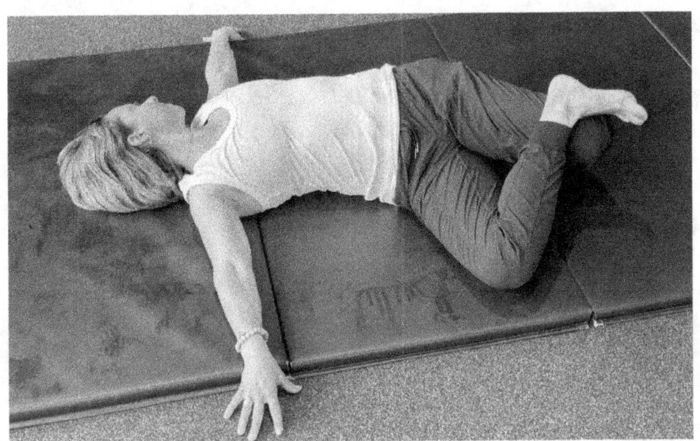

FIGURE 9.11

Repeat this affirmation

"I see clearly all sides of the situation."

Spiritual Mind Treatment

There is one love in the universe.

We can call it God, Spirit, or Life. It is within us and without us.

This energy of love permeates me and casts out all past feelings of lack, being unloved, and not being aware of who I divinely am.

This treatment completely brings back the awareness that I was born of love and will forever be love.

Anything within my consciousness that rejects, denies, or doesn't believe this as the truth for me is immediately dissolved by the power of this treatment.

Together we claim it as so and believe it as so, and therefore, we declare, "And so it is."

Affirmation

"My heart is open to receive blessings."

CHAPTER 10
The Lumbar Region

You know you're getting older when your back
starts going out more than you do.
-Phyllis Diller

The lumbar region is the lower back. This region represents the life supply to the reproductive organs, legs, knees, lower legs, and feet. If you are experiencing pain in your lumbar region, you are not alone. The lumbar spine is the most frequently reported problem area.

Compression in the lumbar spine can cause serious problems. If you suspect your troubles are taking place in the lumbar region, see if your symptoms are in the following list.

Symptoms

Symptoms in the lumbar region usually manifest as the following ailments:

- Constipation

- Low back pain

- Herniated disc

- Sciatic nerve pain

- Menstrual cramps

- Constipation

- Bladder problems

- Swelling ankles

- Weakness and numbness in the legs

- Knee pain

Do any of these symptoms sound familiar? If so, the next step is to identify the emotions that are linked to the pain.

Probable causes

Many emotional feelings can cause lower back pain. These include loss of any kind, lack of self-esteem, and feeling hopeless. For example, lumbar troubles can be triggered by the death of a loved one, divorce, financial loss or fear of financial loss (just as powerful as actual loss), loss of a job, loss of power, and feeling lonely or alone without the support of others.

Reflect on the time around which your pain began. Had you been feeling a sense of loss or fear of loss? If so, what life events took place around that time to cause this pain? Perhaps you lost a grandparent or went through a breakup. Maybe your office environment had been tense, causing a sense of insecurity about your position.

Once you are in touch with the circumstances that have been affecting you, follow our BAM Therapy routine for the lumbar region, found at the end of this chapter.

Case Study: Frances

At age fifty-one, Frances lost her husband, Bill, to an aggressive form of cancer. Throughout their marriage, Frances's role had been that of the homemaker. She took care of the household chores, the children, and her husband's needs at home. Bill was the major breadwinner; he managed the financial aspects of their lives, such as the mortgage and investments, and paid the bills. When Bill passed away, overnight, Frances was thrust into taking on her husband's responsibilities as well as dealing with the emotional loss of her spouse.

If you are married or in a long-term relationship, have you ever thought about the day-to-day responsibilities you would be forced to take on when your loved one is no longer around? Are you prepared for the unthinkable? Have you ever considered that when you die, you might leave financial chaos behind you? These are things we don't want to face or think about; they are just too morbid.

Ultimately, though, death is unavoidable. We are all going to die one day, and the responsibility for our finances usually falls onto family. It is hard enough for those near you to bear the grief of your terrible illness or death without also having to deal with all the matters you could have taken care of while you were alive and healthy. Wherever you are in your health, today is a good day to take the necessary actions to get your financial affairs in order for yourself, your peace of mind, and most of all, the ones you love.

Frances simply didn't know how to deal with the financial aspects of running a home. Within a few months of her husband's death, she had to sell her house and move to a smaller one. She was forced to move on, both literally and metaphorically. As a homemaker and a devoted wife, she faced a double challenge: moving into a new home and moving into a new life alone.

Frances came to see us five months after her husband had passed away. She was in very good health and had never had any serious physical problems. She walked regularly to maintain her good health, slim figure, and general sense of well-being. But when she started packing for her move, genuine discomfort emerged.

The trouble started when she got up one morning and felt pain in her lower back. As the days went by, the pain in her back increased; she started feeling the pain not only in the mornings but also throughout the day. She began to have difficulty walking, bending, and getting in and out of a chair. The pain was even affecting her sleep, and she was constantly irritated. By the time the moving day had arrived, she could barely get out of bed.

Frances's body was physically displaying her emotional fear of being alone in the world and not having the support she had always received from her husband.

Our bodies don't just tell us what is going on; they scream it out loud. The back represents stability, and the lower back (particularly in the region of L4 and L5) is affected when we feel a lack of financial stability. Frances now faced financial insecurity as well as the loss of the stability that her husband had always provided, and those fears were manifesting as pain in her lower back.

When Frances came to see us, she could hardly walk. We started by talking with her about her pain symptoms. In addition to lower back pain, she also had numbness down her right leg. This indicated that she had a pinched nerve in her lower back.

We know that pinched nerves are usually associated with feelings of anger and irritation; and, as in this particular case, when a pinched nerve is located in the lower back, it is connected to a loss, often financial. After we learned about the death of her husband, we saw that Frances was carrying hidden resentment toward him for leaving her alone to deal with the financial responsibility of selling the house and paying the bills. His cancer had progressed quickly, and he hadn't had time to get his financial affairs in order before he became seriously ill. After his death, she had been forced to sell the house to pay off debts.

Frances also harbored resentment toward Bill's doctors. She felt that they had not been straight with her about the seriousness of her husband's cancer and therefore had not prepared her for his sudden death. The person she had depended on for more than thirty years was gone. She felt completely alone and unable to cope with her life.

We began her BAM Therapy treatment by suggesting that she spend a few hours a day crying, releasing, and writing down her thoughts in a journal. Writing things down helps us let go of our emotions and gain a clearer understanding of what we are feeling and why. That alone can bring about a sense of peace.

To assist in Frances's emotional healing process, we suggested breathing exercises combined with a spiritual mind treatment to release the pain and irritation and allow her to feel supported once again.

Each morning, when Frances woke up, she went to her quiet place in the house, closed her eyes, and practiced her

BAM Therapy treatment. The breathing exercises provided Frances with deep relaxation as well as the curative value of positive affirmation (see chapter 5). She placed one hand on her center, or solar plexus, and the other hand on her lower back. As she inhaled, she imagined energy coming in and being stored. As she exhaled, she imagined in her mind's eye the energy being directed into the affected point, driving out the pain and healing it.

Once she finished the breathing, Frances felt completely relaxed and at peace. Then, with her eyes still closed, she spoke the following spiritual mind treatment out loud.

I am Spirit.

The Spirit within me is perfect, whole, and complete.

I am surrounded by a universal goodness that dwells in my body and infuses it with health.

There is nothing obstructing my highest good.

All physical sensations of pain are released and gone forever.

I am fully supported in life and know that all fears are false evidence appearing real.

My finances are healthy, my spine is free of obstruction, and my life is in perfect balance.

I forgive Bill and release him to the highest good.

I forgive myself for any feelings of negativity or anger.

I am happy, healthy, and peaceful.

We included forgiveness in Frances's mind treatment so that she could let go of the resentment she felt toward her husband for leaving her alone and unprepared. We also suggested the short affirmation "I am divinely supported" be used throughout the day if she had moments when she felt alone and experienced fear.

To support Frances's physical healing and help strengthen her body, we gave her three BAM Therapy exercises to do following her breathing and spiritual mind treatment.

First, she did the "finding your center" exercise (see chapter 6). It was important for Frances to experience being strong emotionally and understand that she could provide this feeling for herself and overcome her fears. It was equally important for her to experience the physical sensation of having a strong body, as this can work the other way around and help her feel stronger emotionally. The two work together to support each other, and, when used in unison, speed up the healing process.

While Frances did the "finding your center" exercise, she also spoke the following affirmation: "I am centered in mind, body, and soul."

Next, she did the lying-down back stretch (see movement 3 below). This exercise stretched and loosened her back muscles, helping the muscles support the spine and reduce inflammation (anger). As she did this movement, she spoke the affirmation "I am peaceful."

Finally, she did exercises to strengthen her abdominal muscles (see movements 5, 6, and 7 below). (Note: These back movements also strengthen the abdominals as the two form the body's core and go hand in hand.) Strengthening the abdominal muscles takes the burden off back muscles, which do extra work to support the spine when the abdominals are weak. This helps keep the body's foundation (the spine) strong. The affirmation that accompanied this movement was "I am strong and secure."

Frances postponed her move for two weeks. With the help of BAM Therapy, Frances began to mentally release the grief and fear of being alone. And with that, the back pain started to dissipate.

The exercises strengthened her back and improved her posture, and she looked visibly brighter. She was allowing the beginning of her newfound self to emanate from her core. Although Frances will naturally grieve her husband's death for some time, her physical condition and her spiritual outlook are healthy.

A special gift recently arrived in the form of her first grandson, who was named William after his grandfather. Frances has been given a new relationship to nurture and cherish, and she understands the importance of keeping her body and mind strong and healthy so she can enjoy many years to come with William. Now she sees what BAM Therapy can do to help her daughter-in-law through the sleepless nights.

BAM Therapy Routine for the Lumbar Region

The following exercises and movements will help relieve lumbar pain.

BREATHING

1. Place one hand on your solar plexus (upper abdomen) and the other on your lower back. (See figure 10.1.)
2. Imagine energy entering your body and being stored as you inhale.
3. As you exhale, imagine the energy being directed into the affected point, driving out pain and creating healing.

(See chapter 5 for more on breathing.)

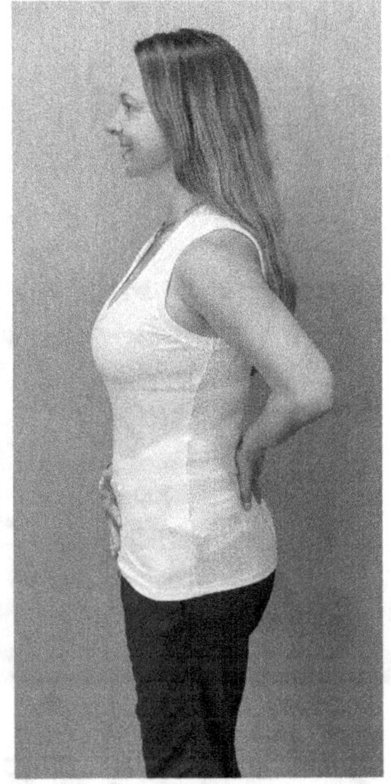

FIGURE 10.1

"Finding Your Center" exercise

Utilize the Finding Your Center exercise in chapter 6 to find your center.

1. Stand sideways in front of a full-length mirror with your legs spread slightly apart. Notice how you are standing. (See figure 10.2.) Is your stomach protruding? Is your back swayed? Are your shoulders hunched? If so, make the necessary adjustments to bring your body into alignment.

2. Developing a strong and firm center begins with proper body alignment. Begin by gently squeezing your buttocks while keeping the natural curve of your spine. Pull your navel inward toward your spine. (See figure 10.3.)

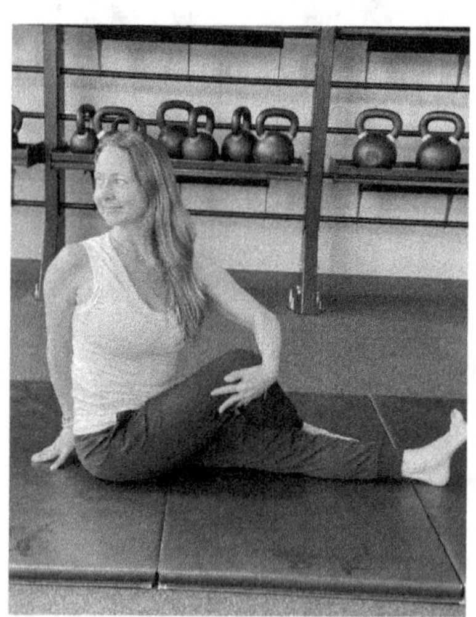

FIGURE 10.2

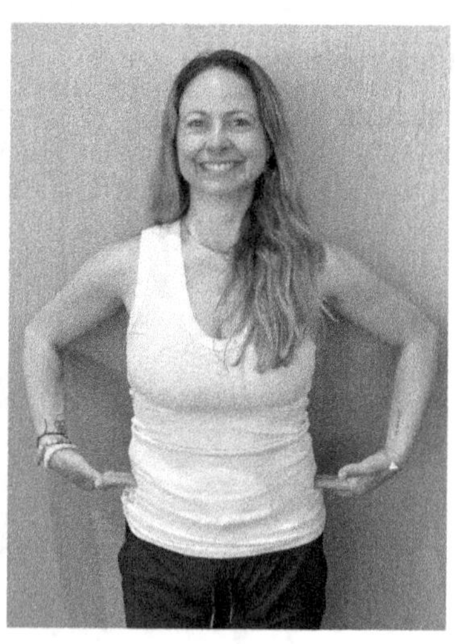

FIGURE 10.3

3. Next, lift your rib cage and make as much space between your rib cage and pelvis as possible by elongating the waist. Relax and slightly pull back the shoulders. (See figure 10.4.) We call this declumping. As we get older, we tend to clump into ourselves, like a collapsing building. The exercise helps reverse this nasty habit, almost like inserting a new leaf into a table.[10]

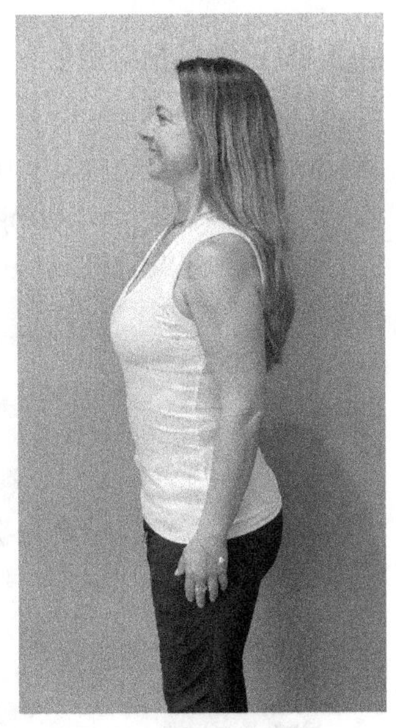

FIGURE 10.4

It is important to experience the feeling of being strong emotionally and understand that you can provide this feeling for yourself and overcome your fears. It is equally important for you to experience the physical sensation of having a strong body, as this can work the other way around and lead to a sense of emotional strength. The two work together, and using both in unison will speed up the process.

Affirmation

"I expand my awareness of my consciousness to include all the good that the universe has to offer."

---

10 For more on declumping, see Risa Sheppard, "The De-Clumping Factor," *Pilates Style*, https://www.pilatesstyle.com/the-de-clumping-factor/.

Here are exercises for mobility and strength.

MOVEMENT 1: BRIDGE

1.   Lie on your back on a mat. Bend your knees and place your feet flat on the floor. Feel your back aligned on the mat, your spine elongated, and your buttocks engaged. Place a small pillow under your head if you need to. (See figure 10.5.)

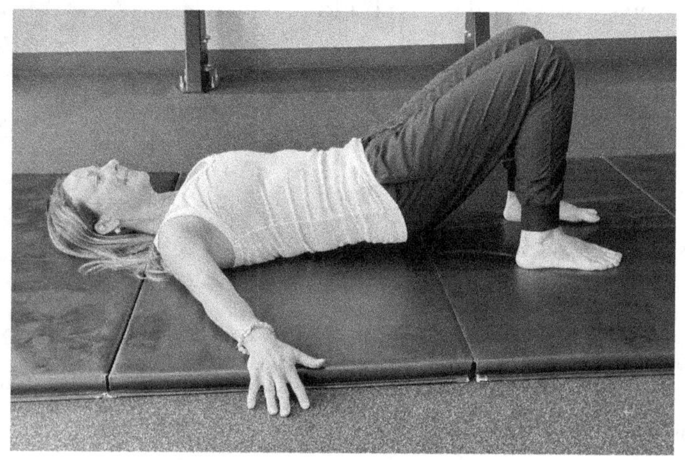

FIGURE 10.5

2. Slowly tilt your hips off the mat, press your feet into the floor, squeeze your buttocks, and lift one vertebra at a time as high as is comfortable. (See figure 10.6.)

3. Feel your lower spine and midback rise off the floor as your upper back stays on the mat. (See figure 10.7.) Think of your vertebrae as a string of pearls, with each pearl an individual vertebra.

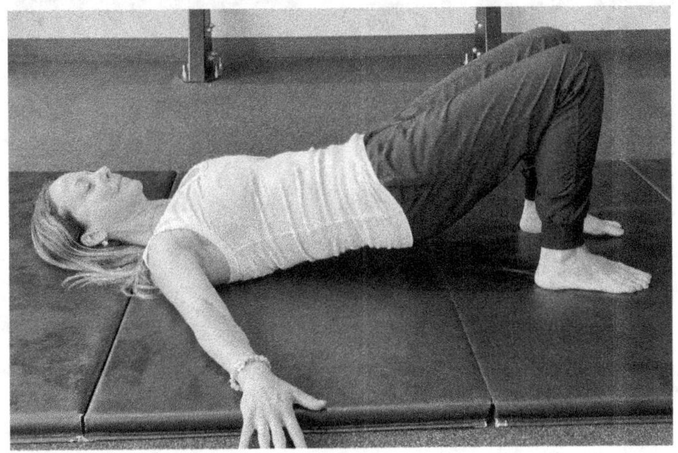

FIGURE 10.6

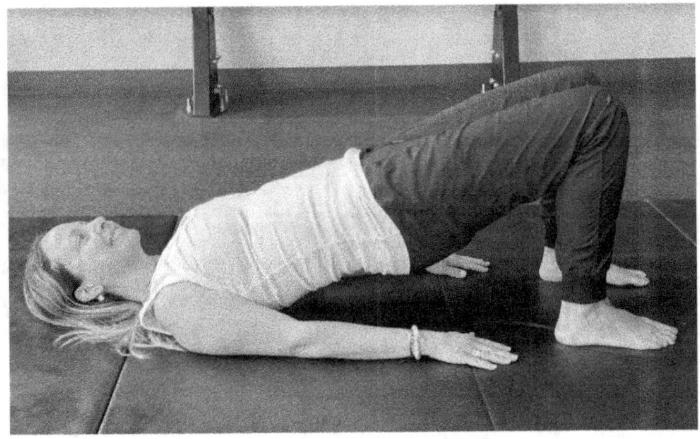

FIGURE 10.7

4. Slowly release your body back down to the mat. (See figure 10.8.)

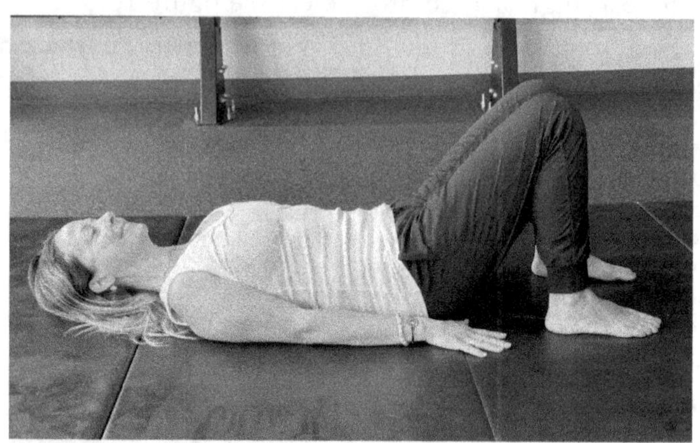

FIGURE 10.8

Affirmation

"I am grounded in my own power. I love who I am."

MOVEMENT 2: HAMSTRING STRETCH

1. This movement begins where movement 1 ends: lying flat with your knees up and your feet on the floor.
2. Lift the right leg up and clasp your hands behind your right hamstring.
3. Straighten the right leg and hold for five counts. (See figure 10.9.)
4. Lower the leg, then repeat three times.
5. Repeat the exercise with the left leg.

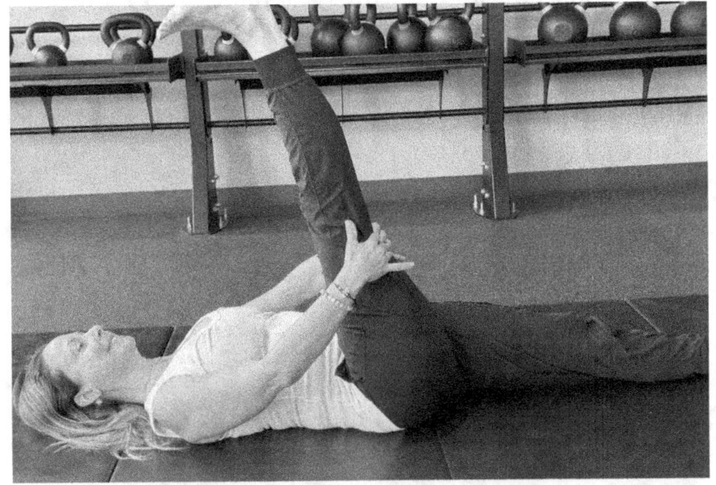

FIGURE 10.9

Affirmation

"I am balanced in mind, body, and spirit."

MOVEMENT 3: LYING-DOWN BACK STRETCH

1. Lie on a mat with your knees bent and feet flat on the floor. Feel your back elongated from head to buttocks. (See figure 10.10.)
2. Bring your knees into your chest. (See figure 10.11.)
3. Place your hands over your shins. Gently pull your lower legs toward your belly. Exhale as you pull. Inhale and release. Continue to pull the legs toward the belly on each exhale. Feel the body relax more and more each time you draw your legs in. (See figure 10.12.)

Affirmation

"I release all tension. I embrace love."

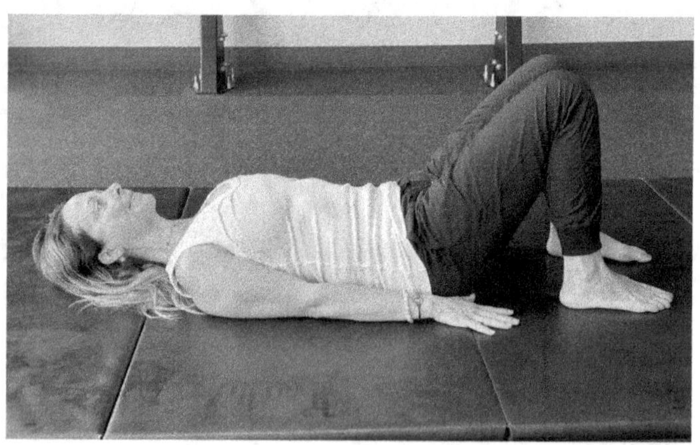

FIGURE 10.10

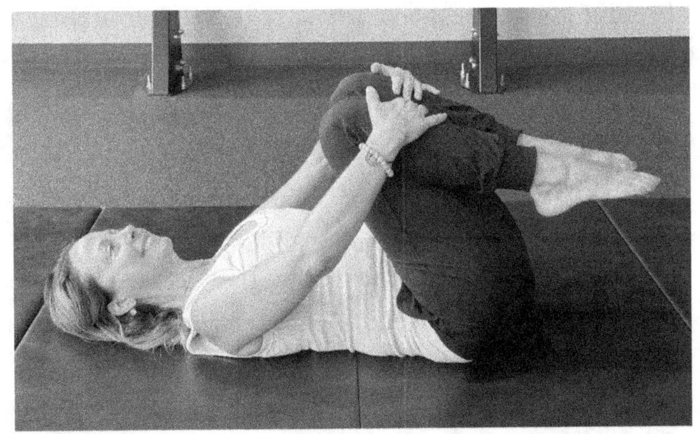

FIGURE 10.11

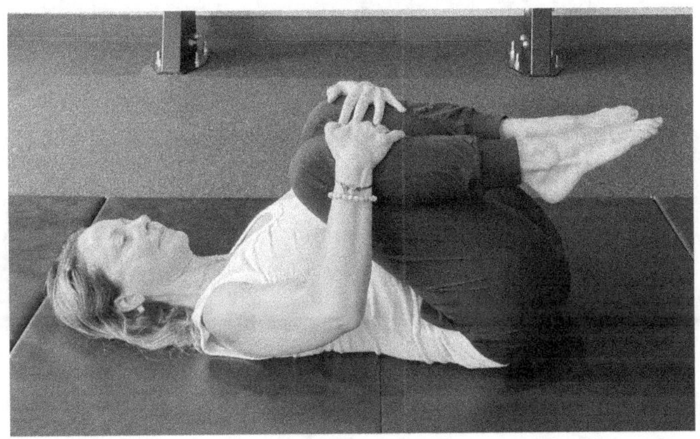

FIGURE 10.12

MOVEMENT 4: HAMSTRING AND BACK STRETCH

Use a TheraBand or a large towel rolled up lengthwise for this exercise.

1. Lie flat on your back on a mat, legs stretched out straight. Bend your right knee and pull it toward your chest. Place the band or towel around your right foot, holding on to the ends. (See figure 10.13.)
2. Gently extend the leg as straight as you can toward the ceiling. Do not strain. Flex your foot so your ankle is pointed to the ceiling and your toes toward your face. (See figure 10.14.) Keep your back lengthened against the floor.
3. Hold for three or four counts, then point the toes toward the ceiling. Repeat the flex-and-point action four times.
4. Repeat with the left leg.

Affirmation

"I love myself."

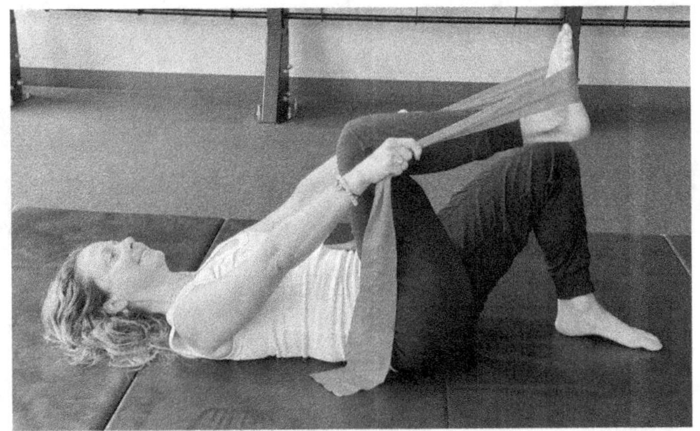

FIGURE 10.13

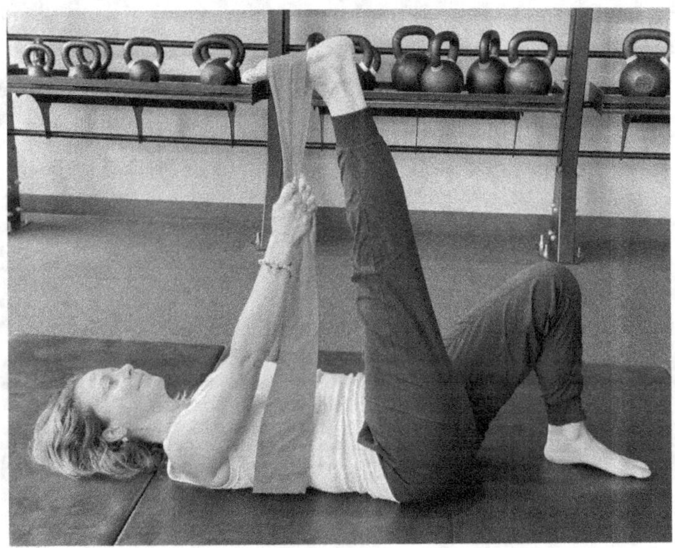

FIGURE 10.14

MOVEMENT 5: BACK STRENGTHENER WITH EXTENSION

1. Lie on your stomach, arms relaxed at your sides, palms facing toward the ceiling. Press your pelvis into the floor. (See figure 10.15.)
2. Lift your legs and extend your arms off the floor, reaching your fingers toward your feet.
3. Keeping your arms and legs lifted, lift your chest off the floor. Reach the crown of your head toward the front wall and your legs toward the back wall. (See figure 10.16.)
4. Hold for two or three counts, then lower everything to the mat.
5. Repeat three or four times.

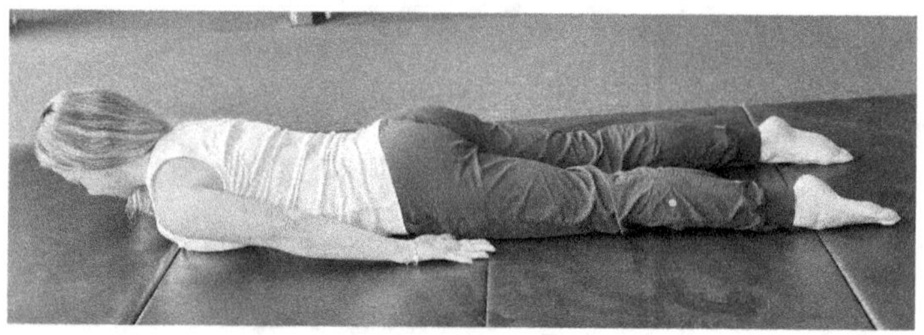

FIGURE 10.15

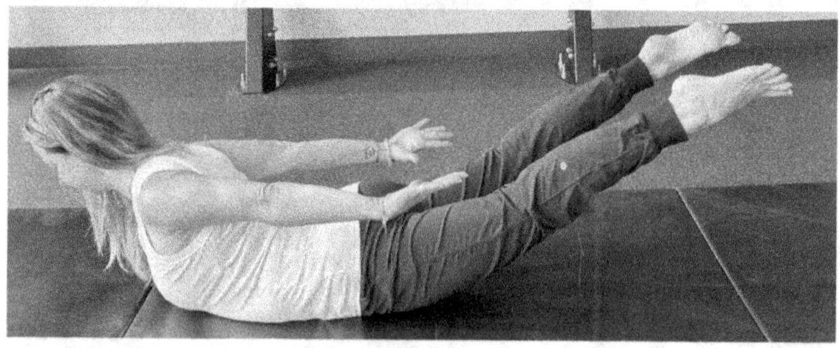

FIGURE 10.16

Affirmation

"I am flexible and strong in body and mind."

MOVEMENT 6: TTHORACIC AND LUMBAR STRETCH

1. Lie on your stomach (prone) with your elbows bent, fingers pointed toward your head. Press your pelvis to the floor. (See figure 10.17.) Feel your shoulder blades open and widen on your back.

2. Lift your upper body and legs off the floor. (See figure 10.18.) Keep your arms bent and your fingers pointed toward your head. Your whole back should feel open.

3. Hold for three to four counts, then gently lower your upper body and legs.

4. Repeat three to four times.

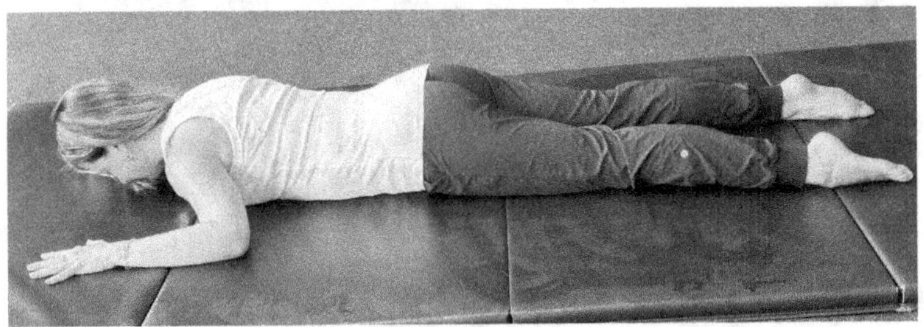

FIGURE 10.17

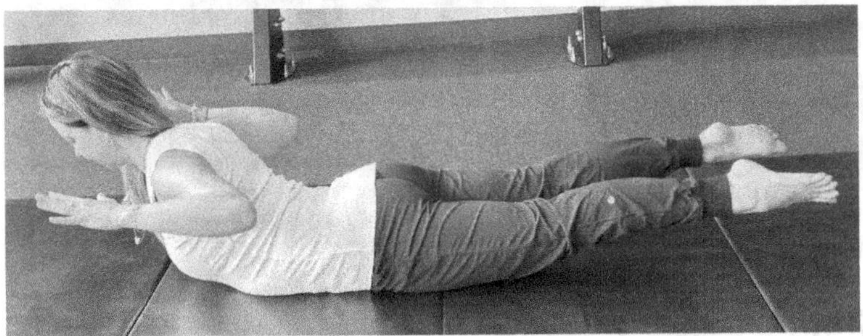

FIGURE 10.18

Affirmation

"I am brave, strong, and grateful."

MOVEMENT 7: WHOLE SPINE STRETCH

1. Lie on your stomach as in movement 6, but rest your forehead on your hands. (See figure 10.19.)
2. Gently lift your upper body and legs off the floor, extending your back muscles. Lift your chest and elbows at the same time. (See figure 10.20.)
3. Hold for three or four counts, then release.
4. Repeat three or four times.

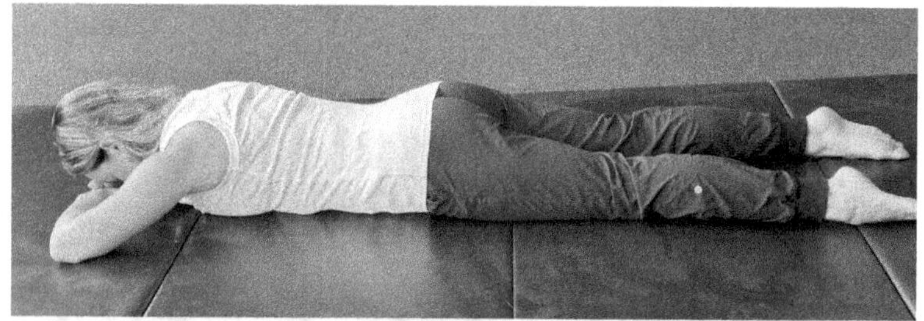

FIGURE 10.19

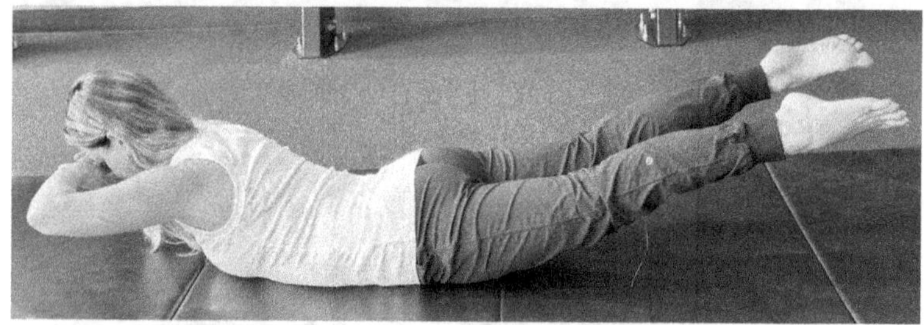

FIGURE 10.20

Affirmation

"My heart is open to all the good in the universe."

MOVEMENT 8: LUMBAR WITH HAMSTRING STRETCH.

1. Lie flat on your back on a mat. Bend and lift your right knee to a forty-five-degree angle. Place your hands underneath your right knee. (See figure 10.21.) Either keep your left leg extended straight or bend the left knee with your foot flat on the floor. Keep your hips stable and even on the floor.

2. Extend your right leg as straight as possible toward the ceiling. (See figure 10.22.) Extend from the center of your body, not the knee. Keep your hips stable and your back pressed firmly on the floor.

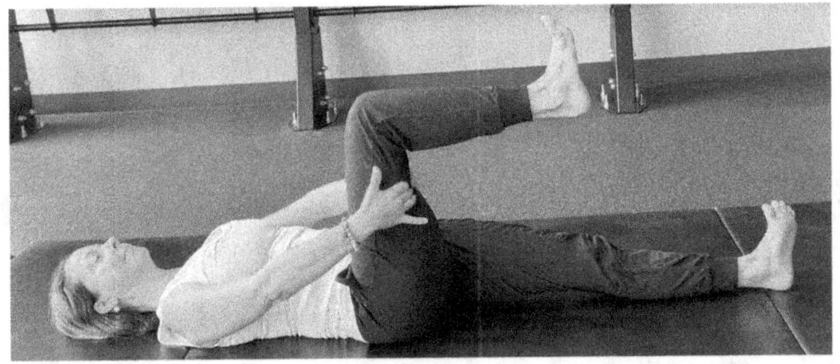

FIGURE 10.21

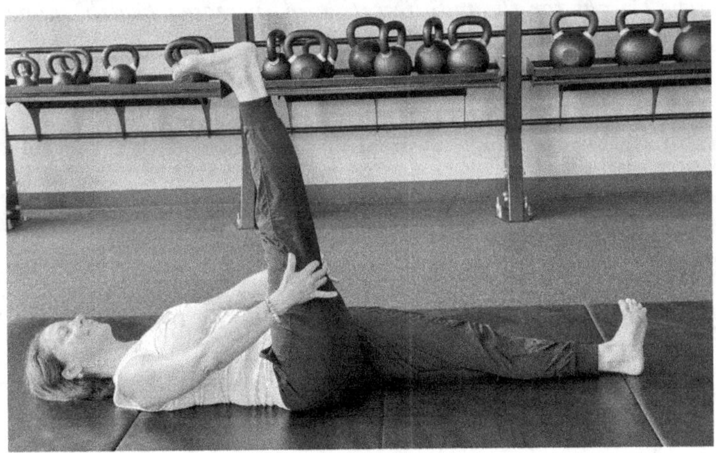

FIGURE 10.22

3. Lower your right knee to the original position and repeat three to four times.
4. Repeat with the left leg.

Affirmation

"My power is limitless."

Spiritual Mind Treatment

There is One Mind, the mind of God, and that mind is my mind now and forever.

That mind is whole, complete, and perfect in its expression, and I now claim that as true for me.

This treatment releases all sense of lack, loss, and limitation of any kind. They no longer have any hold in my heart or mind.

I am abundant in all good things. Money, relationships, health, and creative self-expression are now mine to bountifully enjoy.

I give thanks for the manifestation of increased health, money, relationships, and creative self-expression.

I am open and receptive to a free-flowing inspiration of divine ideas. Nothing can be blocked as I open my heart to the free flow of love and peace.

With gratitude, I release and let go of this treatment to the infinite wisdom of the infinite Universe. I know that nothing in me can negate or delay the open vessel of my consciousness to flow freely and abundantly.

And so it is.

Affirmation

"I am supported financially and emotionally."

CHAPTER 11

Additional Support

Let your tears water the seeds of your future happiness.
-STEVE MARABOLI

We have offered several methods you can take to heal yourself, but there are many additional support methods that will aid you in your healing. The following BAM Therapy exercises may be difficult for you to do, so don't force yourself. However, if you are so moved, do not be afraid to let out your feelings through a good cry.

The Power of Crying

A good cry helps release emotions, and several studies have shown both physical and emotional benefits to crying. Crying has a soothing effect that helps regulate emotions, which leads to a calm feeling while also reducing stress. According to a 2014 study,[11] crying releases oxytocin and endorphins. These chemicals help us feel good and may ease physical and emotional pain. They may also enhance the mood and lift the spirits.

---

11 Asmir Gračanin, Lauren M. Bylsma, and Ad J. J. Vingerhoets, "Is Crying a Self-Soothing Behavior?" *Frontiers of Psychology* 5, no. 502 (2014).

Crying also releases stress hormones. Try letting yourself truly cry your eyes out, and then observe how you feel after.

Journaling

Journal writing is a voyage to the interior.
-Christina Baldwin

Writing things down often helps us let go of our emotions and get a clearer understanding of what we are feeling and why. That alone can bring about a sense of peace.

Kathleen Adams, a Colorado-based psychotherapist and author of *Journal to the Self,* says, "Journal therapy is all about using personal material as a way of documenting an experience, and learning more about yourself in the process. It lets us say what's on our minds and helps us get—and stay—healthy through listening to our inner desires and needs."[12] Adams offers the following tips for journal writing.

Choose your moments. Start at a pace that feels comfortable to you (weekly or three times per week, for example). Plan to write for ten minutes at the start, and use a timer.

Ease into it. Start with a simple meditation or ritual. It can even be as brief as closing your eyes and taking three deep breaths. Read something meaningful to you. It can be a prayer or a poem. Have a calming cup of tea. Listen to soothing music and do some simple stretching or yoga poses.

---

12 All quoted material and journaling ideas in this section are from Kathleen Adams, as quoted in "The Healing Powers of Keeping a Journal" by Barbara Stepko, found on Huffpost.com (https://www.huffpost.com/entry/how-to-journal_n_6479464).

Don't just start scribbling. It will be helpful to have some structure to your journaling. Here are some tips Adams offers.

- *Sentence stems*: Adams suggests writing down the first part of a sentence, such as, "I'm looking forward to," then completing each sentence. This approach is easy, and that's the beauty of the exercise.

- *Five-minute sprint:* To encourage yourself to write, create a prompt to get you started, such as "How do I feel right now?" Then set a timer for five minutes and start writing down whatever comes to mind. Stop when the timer goes off.

- *Behavior research:* Research has shown that when you practice how you will react to a certain situation, you will be better prepared for it. Choose a situation you anticipate, then mentally and physically go through your reaction to it. The more you practice, the more powerful you'll feel over the situation.

- *Springboard:* Adams suggests this exercise to "unhook your brain" when journaling. First, choose a word (such as *relax*) and write it vertically down the page, one letter on each line. Then write a sentence that starts with each letter. Don't think about it too much; just let the thoughts come naturally.

- *Reflect:* Adams recommends spending some time reflecting on each journal entry. Reread the entry, then give yourself feedback on what you just wrote.

This can reveal more profound insights into each day's entry.

These support activities are simple and effective. The trick is to make sure you incorporate them into your daily life. Take the time to not only do the movements and exercises (physical and spiritual) we have given but also use these support techniques, as they will help to reinforce your health and well-being.

CHAPTER 12

A New Path

*No one saves us but ourselves. No one can and
one may. We ourselves must walk the path.*
-The Buddha

We hope the information we have provided here sets you on a new and healthy path in dealing with your back pain. Chronic back pain can overwhelm you and leave you incapacitated physically and emotionally. Our purpose in writing this book is to offer an alternative path to healing chronic pain that is grounded in science and enhanced with psychological and spiritual treatments.

"It is the mind itself which shapes the body," said Joseph Pilates. But in today's world, we are losing the idea and the knowledge of how deep that mental awareness goes. While everybody is talking about mind and body, it is our contention that we have neglected the spirit.

You do not have to believe in God to follow this program. What we are saying is that healing includes being aware that we are full of memories and emotions that are embedded in us from childhood that can cause physical and emotional symptoms. When we do not pay attention to them, we cannot achieve complete healing of our mind, body, and spirit. *Mindful Movement* with its BAM Therapy program, offers tools that allow anyone access to the emotional source of their pain so that they can mend the pain and heal it forever.

There are other tools and other ways of healing pain, of course, but we have found that combining the principles of Science of Mind with Pilates and chiropractic care techniques, as presented here, provides a greater understanding and allows one to let go of specific problems that plague so many. It is possible for those who follow this healing path to untie the mental knots to untie the physical knots, which then releases bodily and emotional pain. We are suggesting that you treat your pain symptoms by addressing the mental and physical sources of pain.

We ask you to consider these body-and-mind ideas to allow the mind to help heal the body and not just use force of will. There is a higher power within you that is there for you and knows how to help in the healing process.

We are always experiencing new and different obstacles to growth and happiness, and even more so in these days of the COVID-19 virus. All the emotional triggers that present themselves to us in this difficult time call for us all to find healthy ways to heal. Now more than ever, we must take time for ourselves, explore, and make physical health and mental health our first priority.

Thank you for taking this journey with us.

About the Authors

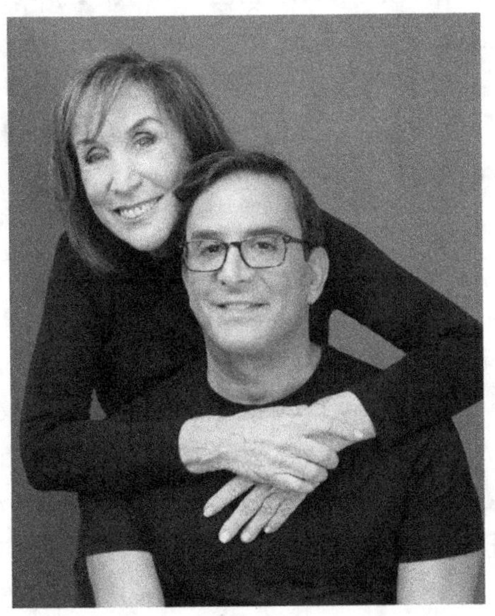

Risa Sheppard is a cofounder of Body and Mind (BAM) Therapy. She has been a leading mind-body-spirit fitness expert for more than forty-five years. She trained and instructed with legendary Pilates teacher Ron Fletcher. In 1980, Risa created the Sheppard Method, an innovative Pilates program that is the basis for BAM Therapy exercises. Over the years, she has worked with thousands of individuals—celebrities, professionals, children, disabled, and elderly—enabling all to develop their physical and spiritual potential. She has been a leader in the Pilates world, training teachers all over the world. She was named by *Los Angeles Magazine*, *City Sports*, and *The Hollywood Reporter* as one of the best personal trainers in Southern California.

Risa has written for major magazines including *Vogue*, *Pilates Style*, and *Muscle & Fitness*. Articles featuring her work have appeared in *Elle, Ladies' Home Journal*, and *Los Angeles Magazine*. She is the author of *Risa Sheppard's Fitness Formula for a Firm and Flat Stomach*. She wrote and hosted a series of fitness specials for television and was a cohost with the late Arthur Ashe on the *Fitness Magazine* television program. Risa continues her Pilates practice in Los Angeles and teaches BAM Therapy seminars.

Dr. David Tannenbaum D.C. is a cofounder of BAM Therapy. A native of New Jersey, Dr. Tannenbaum built a practice in his hometown of Springfield, New Jersey, before relocating to Beverly Hills, California, and opening his private practice, where he has been serving the community for more than thirty years.

At the age of fifteen, David suffered a sports injury and tried a variety of medical treatments. Having exhausted all traditional avenues of health care, he was successfully treated by a local chiropractor. This positive experience was the impetus for him to become a chiropractor. He is a graduate of Life Chiropractic College in Atlanta, Georgia.

Dr. Tannenbaum has treated music icons, professional athletes, and some of the biggest names in the entertainment industry. His outstanding reputation within the medical community for reliable diagnoses and specific adjustments and his genuine compassion for his patients form the foundation of his practice.

www.ingramcontent.com/pod-product-compliance
Lightning Source LLC
Chambersburg PA
CBHW072009150726
47999CB00002B/578